D1571194

Date: 6/20/16

362.196831 ELL
Ellenbogen, Michael,
From the corner office to
Alzheimer's /

From the Corner Office to Alzheimer's

Michael Ellenbogen

Foreword

Imagine having a mysterious illness take over your mind. Over the next 10 years you try to navigate a health care and social system that is not equipped to address what is happening to you. As you slowly lose your ability to think and remember, you have to try to hide the losses to protect you and your family financially. You encounter doctors who are at best baffled, and order a series of nonspecific, redundant, and uninformative studies. And, to top it off, it takes months to approve and schedule tests and appointments. Treatment that might have helped is delayed for years. Your spouse and family are increasingly worn down. Research options are barely mentioned. You get so discouraged that you have thoughts of ending it all, and to protect against that, you try to turn over your guns to the police: they of course say no.

If you want to know what it is like to walk in the shoes of one person with Alzheimer's, read this book, whether you are a patient, care partner, doctor, or other health provider. It is raw and scary, as well as inspiring, given the self-disclosure. As well as describing, sometimes painfully and in harrowing detail, what we are doing wrong, it can tell us a great deal about what we need to do differently going forward. Every individual with an illness like Alzheimer's deserves a prompt, thorough, empathic, and well informed evaluation. Every family needs and deserves support. Every reasonable research question should be pursued.

At the close of his book, Michael Ellenbogen says that, "I would like to be remembered for influencing change…and helping others." I think that he will be.

Pierre N. Tariot, MD
Director, Banner Alzheimer's Institute
Research Professor of Psychiatry
University of Arizona College of Medicine
Phoenix, Arizona

Acknowledgments

I especially want to thank my wife and daughter for their help, support, and encouragement.

Special thanks to the John V. Tucker, Esq. and Oscar L. Lopez, MD, who provided valuable input that will definitely help many people.

Last, but not least, I want to thank my family and friends who shared their time to help edit the book. A special thanks to Steven Gitler, who performed the final edit.

I would like to dedicate this book to my advisor, best friend, and sister, Odette Barnett. She passed away February 15, 2011, after losing her battle with cancer. I thank my brother-in-law, George (Wes) Barnett for marrying her at a time when she was already ill, and then always being there for her. She is dearly missed.

Contents

Contents

Préface

This book will provide insight into the issues I have lived through as a person with Alzheimer's disease. It will cover the years before my diagnosis and the frustrations I experienced leading to my diagnosis.

I hope doctors, business organizations dealing with Alzheimer's patients, caregivers, and lawmakers will read this book. I am hoping they will learn how to improve the quality of life for patients with cognitive disorders. My years of experience with this disease should give others an idea of what they may have to deal with. It would have been nice for me to understand what others experienced and read real-life examples of their reports and issues. I constantly wonder if every new cognitive misstep is related to the disease or if it is something that also happens to the average person.

My name is Michael Ellenbogen. I struggled for the last few years about whether or not to write this book. I decided that someone needs to finally stand up for the folks that are not able to speak for themselves. Please keep in mind that the issues you read in this book are the issues I had. In no way am I saying that you can expect to have the same symptoms, scores, test results, or neurological conditions. We are all different and we each handle dealing with the disease in a different way.

This book is presented in chronological order, to the best of my ability. The final chapters includes a list of tests that are available to individuals who are still searching for a diagnosis and also recommendations, from a lawyer, on preparation for dealing with the Social Security Administration.

As you can imagine, my health history contains a great deal more records than I have included here. I have tried to focus primarily on issues related to my dementia. I speak about my other issues just in case there are relations to the disease that others may also have. While I tried to give you the best description of my ordeal, I may be off a little in my timeframes. I was fortunate that I kept records and notes along the way. Please keep in mind that sometimes I may think something is factual when it really may not be. That problem has arisen from the disease. I do not think I have done that in this book, but it is possible. I do have to tell you that I was never one to make things up, but sometimes I am not sure about what I think is factual versus something that just came to mind. Above all, keep in mind that I have dementia and I have not given up yet.

There is one important message I want you to remember. **Never give up with your dreams, and drive forward until the end. You can still make a difference. Try to advocate for the ones who cannot, because we will be them one day.**

Start by reaching out to the organization below for help.

Alzheimer's Association
http://www.alz.org/

If you need to speak to someone, they have a toll-free 24/7 helpline which provides reliable information, resources, referrals, support groups, care consultation, education, safety services, and support in multiple languages. Call them anytime at 1-800-272-3900.

Chapter 1

A little bit about me/The symptoms begin

Around the age of 39, in 1997, I was doing well in my career. I was responsible for the telecommunications network and data equipment for all of PNC Bank back offices and branches on the east coast. I have never believed that I was of above average intelligence, but most of my coworkers and managers thought I was very smart. I was very lucky to have been able to enhance my business skills, over the years, by working for some great managers.

While most people thought this job was very stressful, I actually enjoyed my job the most when dealing with major issues and crises. I easily dealt with them. Sometimes I would be involved in two or three separate phone conversations at the same time, while I orchestrated a resolution to the issue at hand.

I was always an out-of-the-box thinker and extremely proactive in my approach to work-related issues. I think the reason I was so successful in my career was that I always had very creative ideas. I was also fortunate to have others that believed in my skills. And I was at the right place, at the right time. I was able to influence the direction of the company to their benefit, and over time, saved the corporation millions of dollars. Customer satisfaction was a priority for me. I was also a very good negotiator. I believe that many of these skills developed in response to some of the opportunities I have had in my life. I had the luxury of working for my father for many years. He always came up with creative fixes for repairing TV's in the shop that he owned. I also had many other family members that were also business owners, and they believed that the customer was always right, even when they may be wrong. If ego gets in the way, you may win the fight, but lose the battle. That is because the customer may not come back if they feel you did not treat them fairly.

I cannot say I was a great manager. I was very demanding and expected perfection. I did not tolerate poor excuses or a lack of commitment. I also had difficulty relying on others to perform tasks, because I had very high standards. I had trouble accepting lesser quality work than I expected from myself. Over time, and after discussion with others, I learned to overlook what I considered poorer quality work, even though I continued to find it frustrating to deal with. I limited the number of projects I delegated to others because I wanted to see the actual results. I was very happy to have the power to influence major changes for the corporation.

While I did not enjoy reading for pleasure, I read technical manuals, technical books and many different magazines related to telecommunications, business, and financials. I thrived on being able to find new and improved methods that I could use in my daily life.

Over the years, I became accustomed to the constant changes occurring around me. This skill took many years to embrace. Many in my company looked to me as a key resource when problems or issues arose. I was always the person that people came to for advice with personal issues, problems related to finances, and other problems.

I was doing well financially in my private life. Others have always told me that I am different from most people

4

and that I possess a unique set of skills. I frequently share my ideas with friends and family and they usually profit from my advice. I was always a good shopper for all types of items. I always found the best deals or knew how to negotiate for the best deal.

I always thought I had a great memory and that I remembered everything. I knew the exact location of all the tools in my toolbox. I had many tools to keep track of between work and home. I also used to repair TVs on the side. I was a type "A" personality and could never let things go. I always took care of outstanding issues as soon as possible, even if they were not very important. I never was a procrastinator. I think my mind worked differently from others, because every time an issue or problem arose, I tried to devise multiple solutions to resolve it, or improve the situation.

While I never read the daily newspaper, I did look forward to reading the Sunday paper. I was the person who handled all the financial issues in our home. I addressed most of the problems that arose in our daily life. I ran a TV repair business for many years out of my home because I liked to tinker with electronics. I knew very little about car engines, but knew enough to get by, allowing me to perform basic maintenance and minor repairs.

I was shy and not a very outgoing person. I always had to push myself to meet people, especially at work. I never had many friends and that always bothered me. The few friends I did have moved away over time. My other hobby was boating, and we had a few boats over the years.

Now I am going to go back to age 39, when I think my issues may have started. It was a combination of small things that were just not normal for me. At first, I let it go. But over time, I became frustrated at myself for the following issues. I may not remember a number, forget about a meeting, go blank for some names, and forget passwords. I started to use a hidden mini tape recorder, and a few other things that I can no longer recall.

From time to time, I would comment about my frustrations to others. Many people assured me that it was nothing to worry about. They all indicated that they also had very similar experiences, that it was just a sign of getting older.

While most of these issues are normal when they happen once in a while, in my case, they happened frequently. While most people have what I call a "senior moment," it's important to recognize when it happens too often. I think you are the best judge for yourself and if you feel something is wrong, it probably is. I decided to see a medical doctor and seek help with my situation.

Chapter 2

My first visits to the doctors

In December of 1998, I went to see my general practitioner. I had a lot of difficulty trying to recall examples of the issues I was having. I could only provide 5 examples. He said the same things others said, that it was normal to have moments when you cannot recall things, or make mistakes. I faulted myself for not being able to give better examples of my issues. He was not concerned, but to make sure nothing was wrong, he ordered a number of tests. I had all types of lab work performed, and it was all negative. He ordered an MRI, which also was negative. In January of 1999, I was sent to see a neurologist.

Once again, I was not able to give many examples of my issues. The neurologist came to the following conclusion. I had difficulty reversing an eight-letter word. I had difficulty remembering past presidents. I had poor performance on repetition of the "king story," a short parable designed to test concentration and short-term memory functioning. I could only recall 2/3 objects after a 3-minute interval. My proverb interpretation was quite poor, and surprisingly so.

The doctor's impression, as follows, was based on this mental status exam:
I tend to agree there is evidence for mild encephalopathy, mostly limited to concentration/memory functioning, without involvement of other central nervous system elements. The patient should have an EEG, blood work to screen for B12 deficiency, Lyme disease,

hypothyroidism, neurosyphilis. etc. A formal
neuropsychological testing should be scheduled.

In February of 1999, I had an EEG and the electroencephalography report impression showed the following:
Mildly abnormal EEG due to presence of sharply contoured slow waves seen emanating over the left front temporal region suspicious for epileptiform activity. No clinical seizures were seen during this recording. If clinically indicated, a repeat study in the sleep deprived state utilizing anterior temporal leads or an ambulatory study could be useful.

In March, I wore a Digitrace EEG. According to the neurologist, the Digitrace EEG showed the following:
The study does reveal intermittent theta in the left frontocentral region and intermittent sloe wave activity in the right temporal region. These findings are very mild and would only suggest a very mild degree of bihemispheric dysfunction, though again these findings are not epileptic.

It also showed:
slow activity in the left frontocentral region and also some right temporal slowing, but there were no clear epileptiform features. These changes might tend to argue that the patient's complaint of memory/concentration dysfunction is truly organic, as opposed to psychologically mediated.

In April, I had another MRI with contrast, which was normal.

After meeting with these doctors, I decided to keep track of all my issues as they happened. This way I would be able to provide real examples of my situation. It took me
8

about 2 - 3 months to put this list together. The original date that I have for the creation is 5/4/99, eleven days shy of my 41st birthday. The list below is the copy of my issues at that time.

- Went to use copier and spent a lot of time trying to figure out how to make a double copy.
- Hesitate to dial numbers on phone
- Need to use full concentration in order to listen to choices for voicemail, don't always understand and need to call back to make choices.
- Have problems figuring out what key to push for certain functions on my organizer.
- As I am talking I forget to say some words or forget altogether what I was going to say.
- Forget to do personal things that I need to do like call doctor or other persons.
- When some people speak to me I feel that I am looking at them from far away and their surrounding is out of focus and I have lots of trouble understanding what they are saying.
- Have trouble calculating change received.
- Attend classes and I forget almost everything.
- In class I am unable to repeat back what was said.
- I stare at my terminal and do not know what to do next, at times.
- I forget how to sign on to the computer system.
- I forget my passwords.
- I don't remember where I went on vacation 2 years ago.
- I forget appointments and meetings.
- What is said in meeting just doesn't sink in, especially when it gets a little complicated.
- I think I ask people the same thing over & over. I am not sure.

- I have lots of trouble focusing on financial information.
- Anything that seems to be just a little complicated gets me very frustrated and I usually do something else if I can. My wife was giving me directions to a location and I couldn't understand at all.
- I have trouble giving technical advice to my staff on technical problems. I am confused and don't remember. I was very good in my field for all type of problems.
- Sometimes my staff is late in providing me with things and I am not sure if I just don't remember.
- I read magazine articles a second time and don't realize it until I am in the middle or end of article. I guess I wouldn't know if I forgot the whole article and reread it again.
- I watch TV movies a second time and I have the feeling that I may have seen it before but don't know until my wife tells me I did already see it. Sometimes parts of the movie may look a little familiar. I would never watch a movie a second time before.
- I can't remember how to drive to locations that I have gone to many times before. I just can't picture it in my mind. I was the type of person that you can take me there once and I could find my way back even many years later.
- I seem to get more frustrated over comments on the news or things written in the newspaper. I used to read the Sunday paper every week and I have stopped other than to just look at ads and a few articles that I just scan through.
- I no longer have the patience to deal with issues related to any matter. Return an item, resolve a billing dispute or just get price quotes.
- I have trouble doing my billing on my home computer. Many times I don't know what steps I should take and it seems to be taking me much longer to complete.

Chapter 2

- I couldn't figure out a simple formula on my stocks until someone wrote it down step by step on how to calculate the information. It should have been very easy for me to do. I spent weeks trying to figure it out.
- I speak to people and don't remember what they said.
- My boss asked me a question and I had to ask him to repeat it again because I didn't understand what he said.
- I can't remember things like when I used fertilizer or seeded lawn, within 2 weeks.
- I could not find where I placed a key.
- I never needed direction on doing my job but at times I feel that I need to be given direction on work.
- I was never an outgoing person but I think that I spend less time with people now.
- I am satisfied to just sit in front of the television all weekend long.
- I sleep a lot longer then I used to. I may wake up a few times but I just don't feel like getting up.
- I feel that I am in a daze at times.
- I always had this problem. When in meetings and people speak I would have trouble hearing what they said unless they spoke loud.
- Have trouble with people's names that I deal with often, including my employees.
- I have noticed that sometimes when I turn my head it seems like I see something out of the corner of my eye which causes me to take another look. It seems like a black spot.
- I have reacted negatively towards my employees for things that I thought I told them and then later question myself if I had said it to them or misinformed them with the information.
- Listen to the radio for weather or traffic report and realize 2 minutes later that it was on and don't even

know what was said. I can sometimes do this 2 or 3 times before I actually hear the report.

- I want to get information for the weather on TV and switch to the channel. As I am waiting for report I switch to other channels and realize minutes later that I should have stayed on the weather channel and not sure why I changed the channel.
- I went to a deposition and couldn't remember my anniversary date, month, and year. I also could not remember any part of my work address.
- If I try to compare a word that is written in two locations, I seem to have trouble making the comparisons.
- When my staff speaks to me a lot of times I must ask them to explain things a few times so that I can understand what they are telling me. Sometimes I am told that I'm not listening to what they say.
- I attended a meeting at work called MIM. Information is provided at this meeting that I should pass on to my staff. When I walked out of the meeting I felt completely confused on what was said in the meeting. (I tape recorded the information so I could take some notes)
- I may do something and realize that I made a mistake. I go to correct it and then make the same mistake again. This can happen 2 - 4 times.
- I went into my file drawer for an evaluation form and I just kept scanning back and forth with my eyes but didn't really know what I was looking for.
- I was writing a performance paper which required a social security number that was listed on another sheet next to the paper I was looking at, but I just sat there looking at paper with pen in writing position.
- I asked someone to repeat a phone number 3 times and when I hung-up I still had one digit missing. I was just too ashamed to ask them again because my boss and their boss were there. They did not say it fast.

Chapter 2

- I keep stumbling saying my last name when answering the phone.
- Problems spelling words.
- Can't remember acronyms for field related material.
- When I realize that I am having trouble saying or understanding something, I seem to get worse and my mind goes even more blank.
- I get very frustrated talking to family or friends who keep trying to tell me that they experience the same things and it's not a problem or think they have the solutions.
- Went to a certain room in a hospital at least 4 times and the last time I was going to the room again I thought that I was going somewhere different until I saw the inside of room. I was always able to find my way if you just showed me once.
- I sent bills that require my signature for sign off to my boss without ever signing the bills.
- I make many mistakes today that I would not have made in the past. People at work tell me that I always did everything orderly and was usually error free.
- I worked on a very small project at home to install 3 switches for a sprinkler system. The first time I finished it, it was completely wrong and I made modifications that should have corrected the problems a different day. It's still not right and I must take it apart again. This should be a very simple task for me but it's not.
- At affairs, friends speak to me and I don't always know what they are saying. I can tell that they are talking and I just nod my head as if I understood what they were saying.
- My head feels foggy & disconnected at least once/day. Also experience light pressure just above the ears (temporal area).
- My wife has told me multiple times about a scheduled party at my sister's house that I have asked on what day

it was and I am still not 100% certain what day it is. I keep forgetting it. I think she has told me at least 5-6 times.

- Many times when I talk to people. I start the sentence and stop in the middle hesitating 4-12 seconds trying to come up with the rest of my thoughts.
- Co-workers always used to ask me questions about our 401k or stock purchasing program and I usually had the answer. Today I am not even clear on which is which.
- One of my employees needs to go for training and I remember that some procedure must be followed and some form needs to be filled out. I don't remember where to look for the procedure or where to find the form that I need. (Believe it or not, I couldn't figure it out and then when I finished this sentence, it just suddenly came to me.)
- I keep walking to the fax machine instead of the copier which is nearby.
- I have trouble programming a phone number to be redialed in the phone using the book. I could probably have done this very easily in the past without the book.
- I had a lot of trouble programming a TV using a remote and manual. I just kept reading the same few lines over and over to try to make sense of what it said.
- I am starting to feel paranoid when my boss speaks to one of my employees to perform a task or when my boss sent me a note that said "I assume you already know about this issue"

In June 1999, I had my first full Neuropsychological Evaluation conducted by Dr. Lindsey Robinson. The summary and recommendations were:

Current level of overall intellectual functioning is in the average range, with verbal and nonverbal cognitive skills relatively evenly developed. Neuropsychological testing revealed moderate to severe impairments in information processing speed and sustained attention, with mild to moderate impairments in verbal learning efficiency. Short-term attention, expressive/receptive language skills, verbal and nonverbal abstract reasoning, and cognitive flexibility were within normal limits for age. There was no evidence of clinically significant depression, anxiety, or other psychological disorder which might account for the patient's cognitive deficits. The etiology of Mr. Ellenbogen's cognitive impairment is unclear as, from a neuropsychological perspective, his symptoms are nonspecific. However, the magnitude of impairment observed on objective testing, in the absence of identifiable affective disorder, does suggest the presence of some form of organic cerebral dysfunction. Further neurological evaluation recommended.

In July, I had additional lab work, and all of my blood work came back okay. These were unusual and different types of tests, not normally given.

I do not remember who referred me, but one of the doctors suggested that I speak with a psychiatrist. They thought that my impairments could be related to stress, anxiety, and loss of confidence. I was open to anything at that time. I just wanted to find out what was wrong. I became frustrated from going to doctors who did not know why I was experiencing these issues. I was even more frustrated because my wife and I had to keep taking off from work. At this time, I did not let others know that I was going to all of these doctors. I was afraid that it may affect my job.

I changed my medical at work to the highest paid long-term disability, just in case I was diagnosed with something serious. I started to become very creative in hiding my problems. To address not remembering phone numbers or meetings, I used an electronic pocket organizer.

It delivered an audible sound when it was time for a meeting or phone call. I kept very important information on it, and I carried it everywhere I went. It was hard to get used to at first, because I was used to relying on my own memory. I was either late or missed meetings a few times before I started depending on it. I was very fortunate that my job responsibilities included dealing with all type of problems and issues that arose. I could always use the excuse that I had to address a problem that needed my attention.

Files stored on my PC could be in multiple locations because we used servers in multiple locations. Over time, this became a problem and I had trouble locating all of the files. At first, I found myself constantly using the search command to locate files. Later, I started to consolidate them to just a few drives. As time went on, that also became a problem. I finally copied all my files to my personal PC. I also tried to simplify directory names so they made more sense. It worked for a while, but that was still an issue at times.

While I have to tell you I was ambivalent about seeing a psychiatrist, I made an appointment with one in July 1999. I met with her 6 times over the course of two weeks. I was concerned, at first, using this free program, which my employer offered through an outside agency. I was assured that this information would not get back to my employer, but I had my doubts. I was worried about what might happen if they knew.

It turned out that going to the psychiatrist was the best decision I ever made. I highly recommend this for anyone who is experiencing similar issues. She was able to help me deal with my emotions. She helped me learn not to get upset with myself for not being able to perform a task. I think some of my problems were made worse because when

16

I could not remember something, I would try repeatedly to think about it. She taught me to just forget about the problem, and move on to something else. I cannot tell you what a difference that made for me. She also told me not to get upset over these issues, because it would not change anything, but only make it worse. It felt great to speak to someone and get it off my chest. While she thought my lifestyle and job would be very stressful for the average person, she realized that I had a very high tolerance for stress.

She did make other recommendations that turned out to be helpful. She advised me not to let my employer know about my memory issues. I was very fortunate that I was a manager who had staff reporting to me. She said that I should stop trying to control everything and request help from my staff by delegating out the work. I was not happy with the quality of work they performed, but I had no choice, and had to lower my standards. When I had very important meetings or conference calls, I made sure to have one of my employees with me. In the past, I just went to the meetings and assigned someone a few tasks, with limited responsibility. Now, I made someone else responsible for the project and let them delegate the work out. The person was responsible to get the staff involved and we would meet weekly to discuss the project. These strategies definitely helped simplify my life for a while.

In July 1999, I saw Dr. Murray Grossman at the University of Pennsylvania Medical Center. I was optimistic because he was considered one of the top neurologists who dealt with memory issues. I was very fortunate that he was close to home. Unfortunately, things did not start out well. It seems that every time I go to these doctors, their tests are similar and they ask the same questions. As a part of his test, he asked me questions that others had also asked me before.

I could not think of the answer. It was something like who was either the current or the past president. I watched the news faithfully and this was something I should have known. I could not think of the answer, and I broke down and started to cry. This was the first time this happened to me. I think it finally just got to me and my anxiety kicked in. That is all the doctor had to see. He convinced himself that my issues were probably stress and anxiety related. I understand why he felt this way. I insisted this was not normal for me and that he needed to pursue other possibilities. Luckily for me, my wife is an RN. She offered her feedback on my issues and convinced the doctor to look into my case. He agreed to run some more tests and then follow up with me. He ordered Buspar 10 mg. He also made the recommendation to continue with the psychiatrist.

In August, I had a Brain ScanW/Spect. Here is the report:

The interhemispheric fissure appears slightly widened for age. The distance between the caudate nuclei appears slightly widened for age. The activity in the pons was moderately increased when compared to the results in most other patients and health volunteers. There was minimally decreased activity in the medial aspect of both temporal lobes.

The impression included the following:

The study fails to detect a cause for the cognitive impairment. The minimally decreased perfusion in the medial aspect of both temporal lobes is not a specific finding. It is frequently seen in healthy human volunteers as well as patients with true hippocampal dysfunction.

I continued to take the Buspar for a few months. It was a nice drug, because it kept me more relaxed than usual. I became very easygoing at work. When someone mentioned a major disaster, I would barely react. From that standpoint, I

18

would have liked to be on it forever. Unfortunately, it did not seem to help with my memory or processing issues. I am not one that likes to take drugs, so I spoke with the doctor and discontinued use.

Another EEG was requested by Dr. Grossman, which I had in August of 1999. The impression said:

This is a minimally abnormal EEG because of slowing of the alpha rhythm to 8-8.5Hz in frequency. This minimal slowing of the alpha rhythm is nonspecific abnormality that can be seen in a setting of any toxic or multifocal structural encephalopathy.

In September, I met back with Dr. Grossman. He looked over all the results and he was not sure what was causing my problems. One thing that was interesting, when he looked at my MRI he made the following comments. "The MRI scan demonstrated some minimal superior parietal atrophy that can be seen in a setting of normal aging." He wanted to see me back in six months and to repeat the Neuropsychological testing.

One thing I had forgotten to mention. I used to like to come home and have one or two beers daily, especially during the warmer weather. Sometimes I might have a third. When I started going to the doctors I slowly started cutting back. They all said it was possible that the alcohol consumption could be causing my problems. By the time I saw Dr. Grossman, I was only drinking 2-3 times a week. After meeting with him, I stopped drinking completely.

Chapter 3

Round two with the doctors

It was time to make an appointment for my reevaluation and another round of Neuropsychological testing. I made an appointment with Dr. Lindsey Robinson for February 2001. It was frustrating dealing with these doctors because every time I had to see a new doctor or take a test, my primary doctor needed to okay it. The other frustration was that sometimes I had to wait 5 months for appointments, which was the case with this appointment. The test that I was about to retake was questionable. I was not sure my insurance would cover the procedure, so I had to jump through hoops with the doctor and my insurance company. If the test was not covered, it would cost me about $2,500.00. When you deal with these insurance companies, document the conversation for yourself and ask them to do the same. I cannot tell you how many times they tried to get out of paying, but then they checked their records and saw I had received pre-approval. They kept putting up roadblocks and I had to be in touch with them a lot, when I should have been working. It was bad enough that I had to leave work for appointments, I did not need the added aggravation from the insurance company.

I finally met with Dr. Lindsey Robinson. She had commented on Dr Grossman's findings in the beginning of her report:
The etiology of his cognitive symptoms was felt to be multifactorial, including normal aging, alcohol consumption, and anxiety.

Chapter 3

I have to tell you that when I saw those comments, I was very angry. She was making up her mind before even administering the test.

Her summary and recommendations were:
Current level of overall intellectual functioning is in the average range, with no significant discrepancy between verbal cognitive skills and nonverbal reasoning abilities, There is no significant change in overall intellectual ability in comparison with the evaluation in June of 1999. On neuropsychological testing, Mr. Ellenbogen displays generalized psychomotor slowing and inconsistent impairments in attention, concentration, and memory. In comparison with the previous evaluation, a variable, inconsistent pattern of change was demonstrated, with improvements on some measures and declines on others. This pattern of performance is not suggestive of focal or lateralized organic cerebral dysfunction, and is not consistent with the presence of a progressive cognitive disorder. Rather, Mr. Ellenbogen's neuropsychological test performance suggestive of fluctuating levels of attention, concentration, and performance speed. Objective psychological screening suggest the presence of mild to moderate symptoms of depression and anxiety, and an introspective, perfectionistic personality style. These psychological symptoms are most likely playing a significant role in Mr. Ellenbogen's subjective cognitive dysfunction.

She encouraged me to seek a psychiatric consultation to determine whether a trial of antidepressant or anti-anxiety medication might be helpful in ameliorating my cognitive symptoms. She got me so aggravated, and she would not listen to anything my wife or I tried to tell her. She just did not want to hear it.

After taking the neurological test, I was very depressed for 2 days. I worried that my symptoms were going to get worse over time, and I was not sure of what else may develop. I was extremely concerned about losing my job. I was concerned that if I were laid off or fired, I would never be able to find work again. I felt I could not even describe what I do in an interview. I liked being a part of an organization, where my actions made major contributions to the success of the company. I have definitely done that here, but I still have many other goals to reach. Overall, I think that I have a great job.

I started feeling uncomfortable around people, because most know me to be intelligent and capable of handling any issue. It took a long time to build this reputation. I felt like it was slowly being tarnished, and the people didn't even know why. Since I kept making all these mistakes, I didn't want to end up leaving the job with people thinking I was an airhead. People asked me questions and I had no clue about normal things, like where my daughter went on vacation last week. I made a $300,000.00 accounting mistake. I was having difficulty understanding what people were saying to me. I was having trouble understanding jokes. Noise in the environment was becoming an issue for me. I had a harder time concentrating, even with low levels of background noise. At home, I would spend a lot more hours watching TV. Many times, I watched the same program, not realizing that I had already seen it.

In April 2001, I went back to see Dr. Grossman at the Hospital of the University Of Pennsylvania. He said again that my symptoms were likely caused by depression and anxiety. He also recommended seeking counseling.

Chapter 3

I lost all faith in doctors and was very aggravated and disappointed. Something was happening to me and no one could explain it.

I went back for counseling from May through June of 2001. Talking made me feel better, but it did not help with my issues. I was amazed by the ways I kept finding to deal with my memory issues. I kept finding new tricks to simplify my life. It was my way of trying to survive. It was a good thing I was accustomed to change. The counselor's impressions were:

Client and wife reject the physician's notion of depression as a cause and, although many of his symptoms could be seen in a depressed individual, in terms of affect, mood, motivation, energy, etc., he does not fit the usual picture of depression. It seems that stress, anxiety and difficulty relaxing may be underlying factors.

Around September of 2002, I had one of many conversations with my daughter. I had difficulty trying to let her know what I was saying. I was trying to give her advice that I had given others in the past. I could not remember what I wanted to tell her. Many of my ideas and things I learned were slowly fading away from my memory, or I just could not recall them.

It was ironic that for the last 20 years, I was always the go-to guy for co-workers, family, and friends. We all learn many things in life, but we do not seem to pass it on to our children. Why should they have to learn by making the same mistakes in life? I wish someone had educated me about some of the pitfalls in life so I would not have made the mistakes I made. I did not want that to happen to my daughter so I decided to put together a list of all the things that I knew would be helpful to her. I needed to start right away, before I would no longer be able to remember them. I think this was a bigger challenge than I originally thought it would be. I had to rely on help from my wife and daughter to remind me of some things I had taught them in the past. Some items I could only remember partially, so I had to do research to refresh my thoughts.

By May of 2003, I had created many pages of useful information. I passed it around to friends so I could get their input. Many said this would make a great book, but it needed more work. I thought that was a great idea, and would hopefully be able to help others.

The information in the book explains ways to purchase consumer products at discounted prices. In most cases, the more you would buy and spend on products, the more you saved. My years of experience, and the use of my skills, will help people save money when purchasing cars, homes, appliances, toys, electronics, and just about anything else. They will learn ways to handle customer service issues and receive the respect they deserve as a consumer. People always told me I am different from most people and that I possess a unique set of skills. They have urged me to go into my own business and charge for my services. I now want to reach out to everyone and share my advice.

This information could eventually improve the way consumers are treated, not to mention what this information can do for people. I wanted to live in a world where the consumer had rights again, instead of being treated like a second-class citizen. In today's world, companies and businesses put up roadblocks in order to cut costs. This ends up compromising customer service. These ideas help to break down some of those barriers.

As a part of my responsibilities working for PNC Bank, I made them aware that I was going to publish a book.

Chapter 3

I did not want them to be blindsided if the media reached out to them. Thinking back, there were a few things they did not like in my book. I think it was related to the chapter on banking. They wanted me to make a change, but I refused. I was right and wanted to educate the consumer.

In September 2003, I was fired from PNC Bank. I was involved in some wrongdoing and should have known better. I had been involved with this mistake for over 13 years. My boss, Doug Milke, was in the room when human resources gave me the bad news. He tried to convince them not to fire me, but they asked him to keep quiet and observe. I could see the tears in his eyes, as he was powerless.

My old boss and previous bosses were okay with what I was doing. One of them was doing the same thing. While I cannot prove it, I feel they got rid of me because of my health issues. There were others in my department that did the same thing, and they were not fired. In fact, a year later, I found out from a very high-level manager that many of his staff were doing the same thing a year before I was terminated. His staff was instructed by human resources to stop doing it. There were about 30 people involved. I guess this is how the company can get rid of you when you have a health issue. The can dig up anything when they want to.

Right after I left, a manager at PNC, who was a friend, told me the following story. Someone from human relations contacted him about a good employee that worked for him. They asked for any type of dirt he may have had on his employee. They wanted to get rid of him for one reason or another. It is sad that no one can prove these types of issues exist, and companies like PNC get away with it.

At this point, I no longer had disability insurance and that would become an issue going forward. If they had identified my health problem while I was at PNC, I would have been entitled to long-term disability at 70% of my salary, which was about $85,000.00, plus many great benefits.

Throughout this book I have written about myself and I felt it was important to try to paint the real picture about me. We all make ourselves look better or worse, at times, without even realizing it. I recently contacted a few people, which I had the opportunity to work with very closely. I will give a short intro to our relationship, followed by their unaltered comments.

Joan and I became very good friends over time. We always had open discussions about any topic. I had mentioned to her that I was having memory and focus issues even though I did not know what was wrong. She would just say that now you are more normal like the rest of us. We trained each other, over the years in many aspects of our jobs that we each excelled in. We sometimes worked on the same teams and sometimes on separate teams. While we did not always agree on everything, we got along very well.

Angelo and I were peers and got along fairly well when it came to running the business. He was the manager responsible for the personal computers. We agreed on many things, and also had our differences. But we always worked things out. We interacted multiple times a week. There always seemed to be friction between his staff and mine, but we always came up with agreeable solutions. I do have to say that I was a stickler when it came to following procedures.

Laura and I worked for the same manager and we worked on many large projects. She would handle most of the voice and

26

data needs at the customer end and I handled all special type projects including the infrastructure decisions. We became fairly close and would eat lunch together. Most of the time we ate with a much larger group, most were managers, and others referred to us as *the committee*. It was a very nice group of about seven people who booked a meeting room every day during lunch. I really miss them.

Most of these people did not see or know of my struggles. My direct staff did not understand why I kept doing some of the things I did. I may have created some issues with them because of that and would really like to take this opportunity to say that I am truly sorry. I was told many times that in business you do not make others aware of your mistakes, because that shows weakness. That statement is so far from the truth. Any great manager should admit a mistake and learn from it. Taking risks is what makes us better, and with risk taking there will be some mistakes.

Comments from my past co-workers:

I worked with Michael for many years and, to be completely honest, he was a pain in the ass! Michael was the type of person that remembered EVERYTHING! He was so attentive to details that he made sure that his Telecommunications staff created an (aprox) 2000 page operations manual to insure that the appropriate standards were followed for each possible scenario that they might encounter in a day. He was the type of manager that refused to allow his staff to be blamed for anything that went wrong and could produce the statistics and supporting details to prove that any problem resulted from some other groups negligence!

You can only imagine how I felt when he came to me, a member of a rival team, and admitted that he wasn't feeling up to par! On the one hand I wondered if I could possibly use this to my advantage. On the other hand I thought that he was nuts! His complaints of his inability to remember things as well as he used to were filed under "every day happenings" as far as I was concerned! I explained to him during more than one conversation that "everyone forgets things sometimes" and "It's normal for me to forget 25% of my day - I'm sure that it's the same with you!" But the truth is that it was NOT normal for Michael! He knew that even though his doctors were diagnosing him with depression that he wasn't depressed- there was something wrong! He knew that even though his brain scans came back normal... there was something wrong! He knew that even though he was still more intelligent than I would ever be that - there was something wrong!

It was many years before he could finally convince his doctors that his was not a "normal" aging process. Hopefully, Michael Ellenbogen's legacy is to insure that early intervention is beneficial to the Alzheimer's community. Hopefully those that come after him will benefit from his attentiveness, that his history of early Alzheimer's will help at least one person from feeling lost and alone. Hopefully, there will, eventually, be a cure.

Joan Mears

"Michael Ellenbogen was a hard-working self-starter who understood exactly how to complete a project or support a service initiative, and how to get "things" done quickly and effectively. During our many years in Information Technology together, I cannot remember an instance in which he missed a major deadline or did not serve his customers/users with the utmost care. Michael often completed projects below budget, and many were completed ahead of schedule. Mr. Ellenbogen is a resourceful, creative, and a solution-oriented person who frequently comes up with new and innovative approaches to his projects. He functioned well as a team leader, and he also worked effectively as a team member under the direction of other project leaders. On the interpersonal side, Michael has superior written and verbal communication skills, and gets along extremely well with staff under his supervision, as well as colleagues at all levels. He is highly respected, as both a person and a professional, by colleagues, employees, suppliers, and customers alike.

Sincerely, Angelo J. Valletta"

Michael here goes.....

 I always enjoyed working with you! You were conscientious, courteous, and extremely hard working. Basically, the hard working not only covers how you approached your job duties but how you constantly strove to do THE BEST possible job. Your attention to detail was phenomenal. Plus you usually had a smile on your face and were ready to make the workday enjoyable. I do remember going to a few meetings with you and you drove like a demon! And on those rare occasions when your daughter, Jamie, came to the office it was a delight seeing your "daddy" side.   Good luck and best wishes controlling that Alzheimers...my mother struggled with that as well

Love,

Laura K. W. Silver

Chapter 4

Looking for the next job

I wasted no time trying to find a job. I submitted over 950 resumes. I applied to every company in my surrounding area. I was having a hard time finding a job. While I was still working, many companies and recruiters contacted me offering a higher salary if I would work for their company. I now reached out to those contacts, but none seemed interested. I was becoming scared and depressed because I could not land a job. I was not sure if times were bad or if it was me. I almost felt like I had been blacklisted due to my termination.

The few interviews I did have became embarrassing. I remember going to an interview for a sales job at a car dealership. The verbal part of the interview went well, but then they gave me a written test. The test covered some basic math skills, spelling or meaning of words, and a few other things. It took me a long time to complete and I had a lot of difficulty answering the questions. Unfortunately, I do not know how I did, but I can assure you it was not good.

At another interview, there were two people in the room asking me questions. One interviewer asked me, "What is 6 percent of 8 dollars?" I remember sitting there, trying so hard to figure it out, but could not come up with the answer. I could not even figure out what formula to use. I felt so humiliated and upset that I could no longer do this. I finally had to tell the person that I had a health condition that prevented me from doing that. I asked if I could use a calculator. It took me a few tries to figure out what I had to do before I came up with the answer.

I went to a few other interviews and I think I did well, but then again, who was I to judge myself? I struggled to give a good description of my past job duties and responsibilities. After 6 months without a job, I started to become depressed and began having suicidal thoughts. I reached out to my doctor, who gave me a prescription for antidepressant medication. I wanted to wait for things to get worse before I took the pills. I did not like taking medications so I never took them.

Since I had many guns in the house, I was a bit concerned that I may do something foolish. I contacted my local police department. I explained I wanted them to remove the guns from my house temporarily, for safety reasons. I also said that I wanted them back in about 6 months. They could not accommodate my request. I then told them why I did not want them in the house, because of the suicidal thoughts. They told me that they could take them, but I would have to jump through many legal hoops to get them back. That made it too complicated for me. I had never discussed this with my wife, and the last thing I was going to do was ask a friend. No wonder people kill themselves with guns. The police are not willing to help. A smart police officer should have come over and removed them from me, just because of what my intentions were. I feel it is important for someone to take action to help others in my situation. To give them a place to store guns easily, for a period of time, without the hassles of getting them back.

Throughout this whole time, I was constantly reaching out to my past colleagues, friends, and job support groups to let them know I was interested in finding work. I was also a bit disappointed because some of my past coworkers/friends did not want to communicate with me. It seems that someone from PNC human resources department had said something to them, or their management, about speaking to me. This is what you get after you work hard for a company for over 18 years.

One day, when things were looking worse, an angel reached out to me. My first boss, and friend, who once worked at PNC, reached out to me. Tony Maiuri was a very high-level manager working at Wachovia bank. He was third from the top in the management chain. Tony was a great boss and friend. In 1986, he had given me my first opportunity to become a manager. As I said before, timing is everything. I was offered that position because my direct report supervisor broke his arm in a freak accident. He chose to be out for a long time and I was asked to take over the position. At first I was uncomfortable taking over the management responsibilities because of my good relationship with the boss I was replacing. It turned out to be the right decision. I excelled in my career and made significant contributions to the company. Tony was aware of some of the memory difficulties I was having, yet he was now offering me another opportunity.

The company was going to need some contractors to support a 6 month project. He asked if I would be interested and, of course, I said yes. My attitude and depression changed immediately after that conversation. I saw hope again. Within a month, I was contacted by the hiring agency, who subbed me out to Wachovia bank. This was the first time in my life that salary did not matter. I was just happy to be off unemployment and feel productive again.

I had concerns and was worried because I did not want to disappoint Tony in any way. I knew many people in the department that were past PNC employees and friends,

32

but I did not want anyone to know. This job did not offer any benefits and I was paid $31.00 per hour. I had the opportunity to purchase long-term disability insurance, but I did not buy it. I needed to be in the plan for 2 years before it would pay out. Since my job was temporary, it made no sense to buy it.

When I started the job, I was given many procedures to follow. They included step-by-step instructions on how to perform my job duties. I took detailed notes. It took me a few times to write the notes, because I did not always understand the instructions clearly. Most of the tasks were very repetitive, which was a good thing. I would have hated this type of job in the past. I always liked new and challenging things to do. I found the tasks boring, but I had to rely on my notes constantly to complete them correctly.

After about 6 months, the company began a new project, and my contract term was extended. During that time, I was still looking for a permanent job. The new project was more involved. Ken Kaiser trained me. He was a very patient person. He spent a lot of time teaching me what I needed to do for the new project. I took detailed notes so I knew exactly what I had to do. Again, the work I did was very repetitive. After a year and a half, I was still relying on my notes. I had to give my phone number out all the time, but I could not remember the number, no matter how hard I tried. I kept the number posted on the corner of my PC, so I could see it when I had to give it out. I had many cheat sheets hanging up all over my cubicle that I could rely on as needed. Even though the sheets were located in the same place, I had to search until I found the one I needed. This was very frustrating for me because I never had to rely on notes or procedures to do anything in the past. I actually used to create all sorts of policies and procedures in my past job for others to use, but I rarely needed to refer to them until the last few years I worked at PNC. It was a good thing I had created them for others.

I used to come in to work very early, and would usually leave late. I often put in extra hours, on my own time, because I was trying to keep up with the workload. From time to time, I would hear some of the employees take breaks and spend time chatting, which I really missed. I could not afford to take the time off, because I needed the extra time to make my numbers. I also did not take much time for lunch, so I could get back to work.

I relied a lot on Ken's help, and one other supervisor. I know I kept asking some things over and over, but it took me a while to understand things. I created the necessary procedures I needed to perform the task. I should point out that the department I worked for had a very good database with many detailed procedures. I just had a hard time locating them. After a while, I shared with Ken that I had memory and processing issues, to explain all the difficulty I was having. He was in a position to recommend to management if someone was not doing well, and that person would be replaced with another contractor. He was very understanding from that time on.

The manager in me would kick in from time to time, and I analyzed my performance. I was frustrated. Not just because I could lose the job, but because I would let down those who helped me get there.

On or around November 2005, I put a new list together with the issues I was experiencing.
- Work at the computer at home and every action I do requires a considerable amount of time to do the next function – even for items that I do regularly.

Chapter 4

- Cannot remember my passwords so I created a file for each company that contains the user ID and password.

- I like to read, and find the topics interesting, but can not remember what I read later.

- One time, within a few weeks of reading a magazine, I picked up the same magazine again and read it. It wasn't until I got to a page that I had previously marked with an "x" that I realized I had already read it. This was almost at the end of the magazine. I never did remember to go back and look at the article that I had marked the first time. That happens a lot.

- I can almost never follow the plot in a movie and I confuse similar characters, but I like to watch it. Sometimes I will watch a movie that I have seen before and not be able to discern if I have seen it before. My wife will sometimes tell me that I've seen it already.

- I constantly forget all kinds of things.

- I usually park in the same place daily at the train station and I need to remember the number so I can put the money in the slot. Many times after looking at the number I forget it and I need to go back to get it again. The parking space is less than 100 feet from where I have to pay. I even keep repeating the number to myself as I go so I don't forget it.

- When I have to call and use touch phone prompts many time I have to call back because I miss what the prompts are saying.

- I don't get most jokes any more. It's not even fun to be at some shows because a lot of it goes over my head.

- The other day I took a TV apart that had 6 screws. It took me forever to figure out which screws went where when I had to close it. 10 years ago I was able to take a TV with 25 – 35 screws apart and was able to easily put it back together.

- About 2 years ago I tried to fix my stereo and did something really stupid. I fried it because I left out a step. I never made such an error before.

- Nowadays, instead of fixing things, I make them worse. I totally ruined my daughter's high voltage novelty ball when there was nothing wrong with it. All I had to do was read the power adapter.

- I can not set up my watch any longer because I can not follow the instructions. I lose track of where I was as I go to the next step. I was the one everybody in the family would come to to fix things like that.

- I have difficulty with most electronics nowadays. Even setting up a VCR. I have a stereo that I am afraid to touch because it's so complex to me. I used to be a gadget person, the more knobs and switches the better.

- I can not do more than one thing at once. I used to be able to speak on 3 phones and still do something else without any difficulty. In fact, I used to enjoy it.

- I write many notes so I can remember things and half the time I don't understand why I wrote the notes to begin with. Or I end up throwing them away thinking I no longer need them.

- It takes me a long time to find anything I need in the house. Often my wife has to find it for me. I have multiple tool boxes and could always have told you exactly what box and exact location within the box. Today I'm lucky if I can find the tool at all. Many items I never do find and give up. Some items I repurchase and I later find them.

- It seems that everything I do feels like the first time, even though I did it before. I get better if I do it over and over. I come back days later, or sometimes hours later, and it's a problem again. No matter how good I am, I am never fast. Work is even worse because I have many types of processes I need to follow.

- I spend 2 extra hours at work every day yet my output level is much less than half compared to others. I continue to ask for help and feel very embarrassed about doing so. The questions that I ask are simple. Nobody else still uses notes to do the job yet I am the only one that needs to look up every command, even though I use it many times a week. While I do have good notes, it takes me a long time to find some of my notes and sometimes I am not sure even with my notes what to do. I am running out of resources because I try to go to different people to ask questions.

- At the end of the day I feel so drained and exhausted because I need to think so much and put such an effort in doing things that I am just beat. My brain feels so drained at times because I have to check things over and over just to get it right.

- I cannot learn anything new even though I may read a subject over and over. It just does not stick.

- I try to memorize things that I need to know and can't, no matter how hard I try. Just one sentence is a problem.

- As for math and counting money, forget it. Money takes me a long time to count if I have a lot. Usually I need to count it multiple times. For math I need to use a calculator and usually do it twice for accuracy.

- When we go to a restaurant with friends I try to shy away from getting the bill, and if I do I give it to my wife to look at.

- My spelling is very bad – good thing for spell check.

- I used to be very good at working with people and listening to what they say or mean. Today I misinterpret the information or do not understand it all. I walk away thinking I do understand it but have the wrong information.

- Many people around me find mistakes and are always correcting me. Good thing my boss never sees or hears about it. I have been very fortunate because I am acting as a project manager so when I run into issues with a customer I need to convert I just push the project to someone else. I should not be doing that but I would be completely lost. There is lots of online documentation but I have a hard time following the steps I need to take. I asked others and they say it is easy to understand.

- When I am home and use the computer I often misread what I need to do and require correcting by my wife or daughter.

- The worst part is going to the doctor and they ask me to remember what are the problems I have. – who the hell remembers? It has taken me days to create this list. There are probably many other things that need to be added that I did not add.

- I always think I am right about things when I am not, and I even argue about it. I should know better by now.

- I have become very unorganized because I have paper everywhere to remember things and it is just overwhelming at times because there is so much of it. That makes it even more confusing. My work desk is covered with paper all around and I am working on only one project. In past years I used to keep one or two piles of paper related to a particular project.

- I cannot tell you how much pressure there is knowing that my boss may come to me any day asking why I am not performing when I should be. I know it is not a performance issue but a medical one. I try to give 110 percent even though that may only be 35 – 40% in my case. What do you say? The numbers used are not real but just as an example.

- I worked with one guy doing the same task side by side. In the time it took him to do 10 pages I only completed about 2. During that time I had a perfectly quiet environment which does help me.

- I used to love to listen to the radio while doing any type of work. Now I turn it on and within 2-3 minutes I realize that I cannot concentrate on my work because of the music. Even when the volume is very low.

- In the past few years I do not like dealing with problems or issues due to my lack of understanding issues. I constantly end up giving the other person the benefit of the doubt because I think it may have been me. That's even more frustrating because I was the type of person that would put someone in their place based on the information they provided.

- I just recently went on a vacation (3weeks ago) I know that the boat stopped at 4 islands. I may know 3 of them and that is good because I cannot tell you where I went last year. As far as the picture in my mind they all run together as if it was one place and not multiple islands. Do not remember much.

- I say things that I'm not aware of when I speak and others correct me.

- If I say something to someone and am asked to repeat myself, I will have difficulty saying what I just said. I will be close.

- Years ago I had directories everywhere and merged them all in one area. Today I have difficulty locating information within 6 – 10 directories. Even for information that I use multiple times a week.

- I cannot remember what icons mean on screens like sent or receive email.

- I have forgotten most technical information related to my field.

- One of the most frustrating things at work is being corrected for doing the wrong thing. Today someone informed me that I sent an email to the wrong distribution list. She asked me if I sent it to the correct list as well. While I was still trying to figure it out, she emailed me with the answer. This is something I have done many times before.

- There are many things that I ask others to teach me that I find very interesting. But even if my life depended on it, I could not recall the information they taught me.

- How many times do I need to click on the mouse for information on the PC?

- I call home to pick up my messages and should hang up at the 3rd ring if it does not pick up. I tend not to and have to call back. I am not being distracted during this time.

- Today I started working at work and as I went from one step to another I forgot what I was going to do. I don't know if I am losing my concentration. This happens a lot throughout the day.

- When I go on vacation or have an extra day off, I find it very difficult to do my work when I come back.

- This year I took my vacation and was completely relaxed. When I came back it did not take long to feel like I never left.

- I sent two emails to someone 3 days ago and they have not replied. This morning I sent a follow-up to see if he looked at. I later sent another request to the same person again not remembering that I had sent the emails already twice. I only had 20 emails in my folder of which 4 were for this person.

- My desk at work is full of clutter because I have so many papers there to remind me what to do. Because of the amount of paper, I miss things and they get delayed. When I try to organize things, I can not remember how I organized them so I have to search through everything. When I do that, I find something that I may have lost or put in the wrong pile or folder, which happens a lot. While this used to happen to me before my problems, it did not occur as often and I could usually backtrack my activity and find the documents. No chance of that today.

- When I need to look something up alphabetically I can not tell you where the letter is in the alphabet. I need to say the alphabet to myself and try to match it with what I am doing.

- If someone walks by my cubicle opening I do not recognize them or register who they are.

- Years ago, they asked me how I knew I was slow. It was just an opinion because I could not back it up other than what I thought. Today where I work, my output is being measured and I am way below in my numbers.

    Monthly updated work
    - Adam   11
    - Bruce   36
    - Don   15
    - Hawa   16
    - Judy   17
    - Mike   2
    - Total   97

    Adam is working part time on this project.

- I forget that I have procedures. I forget to know where to look for procedures. I stumble upon them when I don't need them.

- I have trouble locating and correlating information to other information that I need to locate. I forget what I'm searching for and just cannot think in my mind on what the next steps are.

- There were 3 people in the cube next to me and two kept talking. I was trying to listen to what they were talking about. I could not make out anything said other than a word once in a while.

- I am constantly giving the wrong information to clients or lack of information which they point out to me.

After my first book was published, I was invited to speak on many radio shows. I quickly realized that I even had difficulty speaking about subjects that I was very familiar with. I had to keep my book handy during the interviews, with important pages marked, along with a sheet of paper covering subjects that I should address. I also realized that I could not do TV interviews because of my issues. I would have looked foolish, not even being able to speak about the book I wrote. It was bad enough that most people thought that I did not have the qualifications to write a book on this topic, but can you imagine if they knew I had Alzheimer's disease? I would have never had a chance.

Chapter 5

Frustration building, need new doctors

After about 10 years since my symptoms began, my frustration level was very high. It was becoming too hard for me to hide this from others. I had to work so much more than my colleagues did. While I always enjoyed the opportunity to work, it was just too overwhelming trying to keep up. I lost many years of my life, without knowing why I was becoming this way. I have to tell you this is very scary. Sometimes you think that you may be losing your mind.

In January 2006, I met with my family doctor and informed him that I wanted to start a new work-up. I wanted all new doctors to look at my memory and processing issues. I did not want the new doctors to see the old records, because I did not want their opinion to be influenced in any way.

I was sent to Dr. Roy A. Jackel, a Neurologist. I told him that I had seen other doctors but no longer had the records. I wanted him to start as if I were a new patient. He ordered new lab work, EEG, MRI and some neuropsychological testing. The good news was that my new insurance did not require going back to my primary doctor.

The EEG report found nothing abnormal. I had two different brain MRI's. One MRI with, and one without, contrast. Both tests of the brain came back normal.

I went back to Dr. Lindsey J. Robinson, the Clinical Neuropsychologist, in January. She was going to redo the neuropsychological testing. I thought it would be best to use this doctor again because she had a baseline for me and could compare my new results with the old. It would take months for the results. The other issue was that there were not many doctors, who performed this test, that were covered under my health insurance policy.

In May, I wanted to speed up the process, so I went to a Psychiatrist on my own. In the past, a recommendation was made that maybe my issues could be controlled by drugs. I went and saw Dr. Alicia Badayos and her recommendations were as follows, from May 2006:
There is no need for medications and I will leave it for his neurologist to consider.
In the meantime, I could see a therapist for short-term therapy.

In June, just a few weeks after my 48th birthday, Dr. Lindsey J. Robinson finally got back with the results of my testing. Her results for neuropsychological testing were as follows:
Background - Previous neuropsychological evaluation in 1999 and 2001 revealed fluctuating, inconsistent impairments in attention, concentration, and performance speed, and symptoms consistent with anxiety and depression. Summary and recommendations – Multiple aspects of Mr. Ellenbogen's behavior and test performance suggestive of inconsistent /incomplete effort during the evaluation. Thus, this test results described are not regarded as a valid representation of his optimal cognitive functioning. Mr. Ellenbogen's clinical presentation and test are unchanged in comparison with prior neuropsychological evaluation in 1999 and 2001. There is no evidence of progression of cognitive impairments, and Mr. Ellenbogen's developmental history and current test performance are not consistent with a diagnosis of attention deficit/hyperactivity disorder or any other organically-based cognitive disorder.
46

*Mr. Ellenbogen demonstrated an anxious/ obsessive
personality style and some symptoms of depression. His
cognitive can be most parsimoniously attributed to affective
disorder and/or other motivational or psychological factors.*

Diagnostic Impression;
> *R/O Dementia (not in evidence)*
> *R/O Anxiety Disorder, NOS*
> *R/O Personality Disorder, NOS*

Her recommendations – *Mr. Ellenbogen should be reassured
that thorough medical/neurological evaluation on multiple
occasions has revealed no evidence of neurological cause
for his cognitive symptoms. A trial of psychotropic
medication could be considered to address Mr. Ellenbogen's
apparent effective symptoms. He is unlikely to benefit from
psychotherapy due to his reluctance to accept a non-medical
explanation for his symptoms.*

I have to tell you that when I met with her and read
this report, I was so upset that I had made the decision to go
back to her. First of all, during my testing we were not in a
quiet area. Anytime I hear noise, it just throws me off. I have
difficulty processing and concentrating when that occurs.
There was nothing she could do to make it better. I tried very
hard to be accurate during my testing and worked as quickly
as I could. I tried to inform her that she was wrong in her
findings, but she did not want to hear it. I can really say in
this book how I felt about her.

In August, I went back to Roy A. Jackel, the
neurologist, to go over my results. His impressions are as
follows:
> *Obviously the questions at this point is whether or
> not there is an underlying organic etiology for the patients
> memory problems or is this related to other issues such as*

depression and anxiety. We reviewed the situation. Because of their clear concern about an underlying organic etiology I suggested we set him up for a PET scan to see if we can find any clear problems. Depending on the results I would then set him up for an evaluation down town with one of the memory experts regarding not only the cause of his difficulties, but the need for any further treatments.

At the end of August 2006, I went for an FDG-PET study of the brain. This was the first time I ever had this test. The findings of this test are as follows:

There is symmetric, relatively diminished metabolic activity associated with the posterior parietal cortices bilaterally, best demonstrated on the sagittal images. Also, there is decreased FDG uptake associated with both temporal lobes, with the left side demonstrating a lesser degree of metabolic activity than the right, best demonstrated on the coronal images. Normal hypermetabolic FDG uptake is present within the anterior parietal regions, frontal lobes, occipital lobes, cerebellum, basal ganglia, and thalami, This metabolic distribution pattern is fairly characteristic of Alzheimer's dementia.

Finally, something abnormal was identified!

Based on these results, Dr. Roy A. Jackel sent me to Dr. Carol Lippa, a Neurologist specializing in dementias at Hahnemann University Hospital. She had a long list of credentials, and was highly recommended by many top doctors.

On the one hand, it was nice to possibly think I have a diagnosis, but on the other hand it was extremely scary, especially when I found out more about the disease.

I immediately tried to reach out to Dr. Lindsey J. Robinson to make her aware that she may have been wrong.

48

Instead of being open about it, she sent a letter to my doctor about our conversation and reinforced to him how right she was. She really pissed me off with that move. I do not know if she was in the right to even speak to my doctor, because I never gave her approval, but I let it go. This was a doctor with an ego.

I continued to work at Wachovia bank, as a Transmission Analyst, and my contract was extended again. Sometime within this year, my salary was increased to $34.00 an hour. I think my problems were slowly becoming worse. While I used to love working with electronics, I no longer attempted to do repairs. My last three attempts turned out to be disastrous and I fried the equipment. Unfortunately, you cannot make any mistakes when working on electronics. I was no longer doing things around the house. I was easily distracted by other things and by noise. I would bump into things at times. In addition to memory, I also had problems with reading, speech and language, writing, paranoia, depression, use of objects, slowness of thought, anxiety, and reasoning. I am less productive. I was a lot more mellow than I used to be.

I finally met with Dr. Carol Lippa in October 2006. My mini mental state score was 29/30, but I have probably done these exams about 10 times now. My responses were slow and I had trouble with serial 7s. Dr. Lippa asked me if anyone in my family was ever diagnosed with Alzheimer's disease. I didn't know, so I asked my mother. According to my mother, her father was institutionalized at age 54, supposedly for being stressed out and depressed. He had lost his job and stopped taking care of himself. One day, when his wife came to visit him, he was in a happy mood. He asked her, "Who are you pretty lady?" He did not recognize her. He died at the age of 56. My wife and I, and the doctor, felt that he could have had Alzheimer's disease.

Unfortunately, the medical field was not very aware of this disease back then.

Dr. Lippa recommended Athena diagnostics for a presenilin 1 screening, APOE-genotype, and serum protein electrophoresis,

If he has not had CBC, SMA panel and electrolytes, B12 and folate, RPR, ESR, TSH and fasting lipid profile in the past six months, these test should be done. Do a lumbar puncture for 14-3-3 protein, IgG, and the Athena diagnostic panel. Follow-up in two months' time after the diagnostic studies are complete. Consider cholinesterase inhibitors such as Aricept. Maintain supervision for safety.

All additional lab work came back okay with the exception of Folate, which was considered high, at 20.0mg/ml, but that was not a concern. Some others were high, but no concern. In October 2006, I had other tests but had to wait for the results.

I did not have the Genetic testing as it cost over $2,000.00 and was not covered by insurance. My test results finally came back from Athena Diagnostics in December 2006.

ADmark Phospho-Tau / Total-Tau / AB42 CSF Analysis & Interp. (Symptomatic). The interpretation is as follows. This individual possesses cerebrospinal levels of AB (1-42) peptide, total tau and phospho-tau protein which provide conflicting information with respect to a diagnosis of AD. A reduced AT Index (<1.0) is consistent with a diagnosis of AD, 1-3,9,10 but a normal P-tau level is not. 2,4-6,9,10 Please see the comments for further information.

Technical Results
AB42	*190.5 pg/ml*
T-Tau	*178.5 pg/ml*

Chapter 5

P-Tau	*42.45 pg/ml*
ATI	*0.42*

Comments

This analysis detected cerebrospinal fluid levels of AB(1-42) peptide, total tau and phospho-tau protein which provide conflicting information with respect to a diagnosis of AD. Reduced AB(1-42) and increased total tau levels, leading to an AT index of less than 1.0 differentiate AD from non-AD patients with a specificity of 83-89%, 1-3 but the majority of AD patients would also tend to have elevated P-tau levels (>61 pg/ml) which were not found in this analysis. 2,4,5,6 the combined result therefore is not completely consistent with a diagnosis of AD, although some AD patients do fall in this range of biomarkers. This combination of biomarker values might be indicative of non-AD dementia (particularly FTD and DLB), since these causes of dementia are much more likely to have a normal P-tau concentrations (< 61 pg/ml). Other cause of this individuals symptoms cannot be excluded. Therefore, these test results must be interpreted in the context of clinical findings and other laboratory data.

On or around July 2007, I was sent for another round of Neuropsychological testing, with a new doctor. This would be my fourth test, so by now I had many baselines established on my performance. I went to Dr. Sandra P Koffler, at Drexel University College of Medicine.

I started to investigate the possibility of going out on disability. As I performed my research, I became concerned and aggravated. I spoke to about 8 or 10 different people. Their organizations dealt with issues related to memory and the eligibility for Supplemental Security Income (SSI). They all told me this would be hard to prove, especially since they cannot see physical problems. They recommended getting a lawyer from the start. One of these people was very high level within the Social Security Administration.

During this time, I had an interest to drive a motorcycle. I was having difficulty trying to learn the manual for the test. I would read the data, but could not recall what I read hours later. I finally gave up. I also had an issue where I forgot to pay my real estate taxes. This was now about the third financial mistake I made in the last year. Previous mistakes involved paying the wrong credit cards. It was definitely becoming apparent that I may not be able to handle the financial responsibilities much longer. I even spent extra time to ensure I was accurate, but that didn't help. I made more mistakes this year than I made in my lifetime in regard to financial issues. I started having intermittent minor vision problems. I would see ghost images when looking at printed material. It did not matter if it was large or small print. I also saw ghosting, at times, when I looked at wall corners or ceiling panels.

My report from Dr. Sandra P Koffler was completed October 1, 2007. Her summary states:

Mr. Ellenbogen's performances on the various test of memory were, at times, consistent with recognized neurobehavioral correlates to temporal and parietal lobe dysfunction, but not consistently so. Mr. Ellenbogen's demonstrated significant impairments in the domains of learning and memory, primarily for verbal information. Current results indicating possible worsening of his verbal memory provide a basis for considering of a neurological disorder, i.e. mild cognitive impairment. Conversely, visuospatial, visual motor, and constructional abilities remained intact, and generally improved which would not be expected.

Chapter 5

Impressions:
1. *Mild Cognitive Impairment*
2. *Emotional Disturbace*
   a. *R/O Anexity Disorder*
   b. *R/O Dysthymic v. Depressive Disorder*
   c. *R/O Obsessive-Compulsive Personality Disorder*
3. *R/O Remote Effects of Prior Head Injury (unlikely)*

At work, I was given notice that my contract would end by December 2007. I reached out to a few lawyers and they suggested getting examples of my work from my peers. I reached out to the person I worked most closely with through the following letter.

Hi Ken,

I am following up in reference to my conversation with you from a few weeks ago, about issues you noticed while I worked at Wachovia. Please include all things you can think of whether it is good or bad. How did I perform my job? Did you help me at all? Did you notice any memory or other problems? I need you to be extremely honest with me no matter how bad things may be. The reason I am requesting this is because I am concerned that no one else sees my issues and they all think I'm doing a great job, when in reality it's your assistance that is keeping me afloat. This may help me in the future and it is very important to me should I ever need to apply for disability. Thanks

Below is Ken's response.

Mike,

I had already started working on it and it took longer then I thought it would. First of all, I want to let you know that I do not feel comfortable doing this. Keep in mind that you asked me for the honest truth. I really like you as a friend and I don't want my comments to jeopardize our friendship. I'm doing this to help you.

You were extremely slow in picking things up when you first started in March of 2004. There are many things that others learn within 2-3 months that you still don't haven't grasped. Simple commands that you use daily still need to be looked up using your long list of notes. You are very slow in processing information and many times you just don't seem to understand what I'm saying unless I explain it multiple times and in different ways. You make mistakes frequently. And from what I can see you still can't remember your work phone number even though you repeat it daily. You were always willing to help others no matter what, even if you were unsure of the solution.

You told me about your memory problems but I tried to overlook these issues and offer encouragement. At first I just thought you were like me. I forget things all the time but I think that is normal for my age. Over time I have come to realize how serious your problem really is. When I stood behind you, waiting for you to perform tasks, I tried to be patient. But it took you so long to figure things out that I jumped in, to direct you to the next step, which did not always help. Often I just did the work for you, because it was quicker for me to do the work than to wait for you to do it. I don't think you are much worse than when you started, but I do think you have declined some. It's hard to tell.

54

It's a good thing we became good friends. Many contract workers who started after you were terminated for not meeting the job requirements. I probably trained you 8 times longer than any other person and you continue to need my help till this day. I know you also went around asking the rest of the staff for help. There were many times you have asked the same questions over and over.

I don't know how, but somehow you always managed to find a way around the system without my help. While your numbers were always lower, you found a way to associate yourself with other tasks. You gave clients 3 options instead of 9 to keep the conversion simple. Even with all of that that your numbers were still not up to par. Every time you got in a jam with a transmission, luck was on your side, and you were able to pawn it off to someone else. You were much worse off when overwhelmed or under pressure, things came to a halt. I had to allow you to move at your own pace.

If it weren't for your past reputation and knowing some of the senior management, I would not have taken a liking to you. I could tell that you were always trying very hard. You worked 1 ½ hours extra every day, just trying to keep up. I also knew you did not mingle with the rest of us on breaks just so you could make higher numbers. I think I am rambling on too long. Let me know if this is okay. I wish you the best of luck wherever you go and I hope the doctors figure out what's causing your cognitive problems. It truly was a pleasure to work with you as a friend.

I remember having difficulty each year with a compliance questionnaire that had to be completed. It was mandatory to take the test and get a passing grade. It was getting harder and harder for me as each year passed. This was an educational class given on the computer. You could take this test any time within a 2-month period, in private. This last year I took the test and failed it badly. The next day, I came in very early before anybody in my department was in. I started taking the test again. This time I took snapshots of every screen so I could go back and look at the information. Now I had an electronic file to go through to search for the answers. This test was fairly easy for me about 7 years ago. With all the cheating this time, I only just passed it. That was kind of scary.

In October 2007, I met again with Dr. Carol Lippa to go over my findings. Her impression now changed to Mild Cognitive Disorder. She was not planning any type of treatment until my wife and I pushed the issue. She then discussed the benefits of treating me for psychiatric versus organic etiologies. Since my wife and I both felt strongly that there was not a psychiatric etiology, she decided to treat me for Alzheimer's disease. Aricept was initiated at a dose of 5mg a day. She also continued to request that I have the presenilin 1 and APOE genotype testing. She wanted me to follow-up in 3 months.

While I wanted to take the genotype testing, I did not because of the cost. The test would not definitely indicate that I had Alzheimer's, unless I had the gene. Others that did not have the gene may still get Alzheimer's. I decided against taking this test based on the possible benefits and cost.

Chapter 6

Is it really Alzheimer's

It was December 2007, at the age of 49, when my job ended. As I was leaving, I tried to find out what my coworkers had felt about my performance during my 4 years at Wachovia. It seems that I did a good job, because they had no clue that I was having difficulties. I guess it was worth all the extra effort I put in to get the job done. I felt burned out, even though the job should have been easy to do. I applied for unemployment compensation while I continued to look for a new job. I had never stopped looking for a job, even while I was working.

My wife and I would disagree every time I saw a possible opportunity for a high-level position. She did not believe I could handle that type of position anymore and was concerned I would run the company into the ground. I still thought, if I had good people working around me, I could delegate the work and use my skills to make a difference overseeing the department. To tell you the truth, I was not sure I could still do it, but I wanted a last shot to try. At one time, I was a workaholic, so giving up was not in my nature. I had come to a point where I enjoyed the power to influence changes in organizations that lead to improvements to financials and service. I realized that I could no longer make a decision on the spot, but with added time, I still came up with some good solutions. The solutions may not have been as good as they once were, but as someone once said to me, "While you may have memory problems, you are now at the same level as the average person." I had one or two interviews that I do not think went well.

I finally reached out to a lawyer who specialized in medical disability cases. He felt my case was going to be a tough one. He recommended that I see doctors for every health issue I had, because that would be helpful in qualifying for disability. While I did not feel comfortable doing that, I definitely had many health issues that I suffered from on a daily basis. I started making appointments with all of the different doctors.

In early March of 2008, my lawyer submitted my application for disability. Even though I applied for disability, I was still hoping it would not come to that. I kept doing everything I could to try to secure a job. One of my major concerns in not delaying my application was the determination of how much I could collect. The longer I waited to file for SSI, the less I could receive monthly once I was eligible. Remember, my salary was a lot less when I went to Wachovia. They figure out your monthly disability payment based on the last 5 full quarters that you worked and received a salary. That same figure is used to determine your retirement benefit.**

The lawyer's fees are limited to $5,300.00 by the Social Security Administration. The lawyer does have the right to charge for additional expenses, such as expert witnesses if needed, postage, fees for doctors' records, etc. If you do not have all of your medical records, the Social Security Administration can obtain them. They must provide you a copy when they make a decision. It is best to get your own records because most doctors will not charge you. Do not tell them it is for your case. Tell them that you want the records for your home file. You are entitled to one copy that you should maintain at home. I advise keeping them on a computer so you can send them out electronically, without the cost of copies and postage. If the lawyer requests records from the doctor, he may be charged between $25.00 to $200.00, depending on what is involved.

According to the Social Security Administration, it does not matter how much you earned before you became ill. If they can find a job that you are able to do, you must take it, even if it pays significantly less. At one point, I was told that SSI could have me collecting tickets at a movie theater. I think I would have gone crazy if I were assigned a job like that. Also, keep in mind my salary would be much lower than if I collected SSI. I cannot tell you how scary it was to think that could be possible after performing such a high-level job for all those years. The system really needs to be changed. Luckily for me, I had other health issues that prevented me from standing for a long time.

In March of 2008, I had another MRI without contrast. The result was normal and showed no change from January 2006. I was sent for another neuropsychological evaluation, which I had in May 2008, eight days before my 50th birthday. I met with Dr. David J. Libon, a neurologist at Drexel University College of Medicine. I expected to have improved, because I had been taking Aricept. I left Dr. Libon's office with a different feeling, because I felt I scored worse. Until now, the neuropsychological evaluations were all about the same. In fact, I think they may have even been the same questions in many cases. It seems that this time, the testing was very different. As soon as the doctor realized I was struggling with something, he would take a different approach. Many of the things I did seemed different. Another problem I ran into was that it was noisy in the room. As soon as I complained, he moved the test to his own personal office across the street.

Around this same time, I was going to try a new drug in place of the Aricept. The Aricept was making me feel sick every day until about 2 PM. It was also making me have many active thoughts throughout the night, sometimes interfering with my sleep. Before I started taking Aricept, I never used to eat breakfast. Afterward I purposely forced myself to eat to eliminate the feeling of nausea. It did help some. I tried to switch to Exelon. The first time I took that drug, I became very ill after 1 hour. I felt very hot and was dizzy and nauseous. I had numbness in my fingers that spread to my arms and chest. I was alone in the house and called the police to stay with me until my wife could get home from work. According to the police and medic, that responded, I was "gray" when they arrived. I started to feel a little better after I vomited the medicine. After that episode, I went back to the Aricept.

In June, I received a request to see two doctors selected by the Bureau of Disability Determination. One doctor was going to perform a Physical Examination, the other was going to do neuropsychological testing. After my visits to them, both of these doctors were in agreement with my doctor's findings, and in my favor. What I really found interesting is that the person in the Social Security office responsible for determining my eligibility for Social Security, who never met me, disagreed with many of the findings. This person even disagreed with the findings of their own doctors' recommendations.

The Social Security Administration replied with the following:

We determined that your condition is not severe enough to keep you from working. We considered the medical and other information, your age, education, training, and work experience in determining how your condition affects your ability to work.

Chapter 6

They gave me 60 days to file an appeal if I disagreed with their findings. My lawyer filed for the appeal.

I really found it frustrating that they did not have many of my recent medical records. How are they supposed to do a fair job if they do not even have the most recent records? It is sad that these people do this job and put up all kinds of roadblocks for people who really need the help. Over the course of the last few months, I had discussions with many people who know someone on disability insurance. Most were not even in need, but they were collecting. As one person told me, it all depends on who you know. I think there is something wrong with this system. If I were a low-level person, I probably would have been approved immediately. This is what you get for trying to be a better person in this world. You are penalized.

Dr. David J. Libon's neuropsychological evaluation results were available in June. His Summary and diagnosis are as follows:

Michael Ellenbogen is a middle-aged man who was referred for a neuropsychological evaluation because of suspected dementing illness. The patient gives a 10-year history of cognitive decline including difficulty maintaining employment. On the basis of the patient's self description a primary progressive aphasia appears to be present. Mr. Ellenbogen described increasing word finding, comprehension, writing and spelling difficulty.

Today's evaluation verifies the patient's self-report. Performance on all language related tests was quite impaired. Conversational speech was positive for mild word finding difficulty. Word finding difficulty was also seen on formal tests requiring the patient to name pictures and define words etc. Performance on tests that assess comprehension was quite impaired considering the patient premorbid occupational history. Spelling and writing problems were also noted. Mr. Ellenbogen also displayed problems on selected tests that assess executive control and working memory. The verbal nature of these test contributed to his difficulty. Problems were also seen on verbal memory test were a primary amnesia is present.

By contrast, the patient performed very well on visuospatial test such as when asked to produce clock drawings and copy the Rey Complex Figure. Visual memory, as assess with immediate and delayed recall of the Rey Complex Figure, was intact. In sum, the profile obtained today suggests the presence of an emerging semantic dementia. A summary of test scores is listed below.

Domain of Cognitive Function

Attention/ Short-Term Storage and Rehearsal
Automatized Mental Control   +0.53
 Digits Backwards (rehearsal/ storage)   +0.10
(Mean Composite Index)   **(z= +0.31; 62nd percentile)**

Working Memory
Complex Mental Sets (mental control)   -1.57
Digits Backwards (manipulation)   +0.24
(Mean Composite Index)   **(z= -.0.66; 25th percentile)**

Executive Control
Letter Fluency('F,A,S')   -1.50
Trail Making – Part B   -2.10
(Mean Composite Index)   **(z= -1.80; 4th percentile)**

Information Processing Speed/
Digit Symbol   -1.66
Trail Making – Part A   -1.00
(Mean Composite Index)   **(z= -1.33; 9th percentile)**

General Intellectual Functioning
WAIS-III Information   -0.66

WAIS-III Similarities	*-0.66*
WAIS-III Vocabulary	*-1.00*
(Mean Composite Index)	***(z= -0.73; 23rd percentile)***

Language/ Semantic Knowledge
Naming/ Lexical Retrieval (BNT)	*-1.68*
Lexical Knowledge ('animal' WLG)	*-1.90*
Verbal Concept Formation	
(Mean composite Score)	***(z= -1.79; 4th percentile)***

Memory and Learning (PrVLT)
Delay free recall	*-1.16*
Cue Recall Intrusions	*-0.18*
Delayed Recognition	*-4.65*
(Mean Composite Index)	***(z= -1.99; 2nd percentile)***

Diagnosis *– semantic dementia*

Treatment Plan/ Recommendations

Present & Future Living Situation
1.)   A mild to moderate level of supervision is recommended to monitor the patient's compliance with the patient's medication regime and everyday activities.

Driving
1.)   A driving evaluation should be considered.

Competencies
1.)   Mr. Ellenbogen is fully able to make very routine decisions. However, the assistance of a family member is necessary in order for the patient to make complex decision regarding financial matters. In this regard the patient and family should consider consulting an attorney to discuss drawing up a living will, power of attorney, and related issues.

Activities of Daily Living

1.)   In order to facilitate the patient's independence, everyday tasks should be made routine. Also, wherever possible, Mr. Ellenbougen should rely on past knowledge. For example, the patient might have comparatively little difficulty preparing a meal with familiar utensils and ingredients in a familiar environment. However, tasks requiring the use of newly learned information, or in situations that are not familiar will be more problematic.

2.)   The patient should be encouraged to perform only one task at a time, and the patient should not be interrupted while performing activities. It will be more difficult for the patient to perform activities of daily living if engaged in conversation. In addition, environmental distractions (e.g., television, radio, etc.) should be kept at a minimum to allow the proper focus to complete the task at hand.

Language and Communication
1.)   The family must not assume that the patient comprehends what is being said. Just as one can repeat a phrase in a foreign language, but not know the meaning of the words, dementia patients may be capable of repeating verbal information even when the meaning of words is lost. It is important that the family does not assume that the patient comprehends information just because a phrase or sentence can be repeated.

2.)   In an attempt to facilitate the comprehension of everyday conversation, caretakers should speak in simple sentences. Gestures and exaggerated prosody may also increase the patient's comprehension.

Further Diagnostic and Treatment Services
1.)   A trial of medication designed to treat the patient's memory disorder should be considered.

Chapter 6

2.)   *The patient's depression should be monitored.*

In June 2008, I again met with Dr. Carol Lippa to go over the findings. Her diagnosis now changed to Semantic dementia in a gentlemen with mild posterior atrophy. Her recommendations included the following:

Recommend a driver safety evaluation at Moss Rehab if Mr. Ellenbogen wishes to drive. Follow-up with Dr. Libon to review what types of employment might be realistic. Mr. Ellenbogen wishes to do a professional job. His neuropsychological testing profile, overall, suggests that he might not be successful at this. Send records to Dr. Jordan Grafman at the NIH to determine whether he would be a candidate for clinical trials. Maintain supervision for safety to be sure that no safety-related issues develop. His wife seems realistic about this.

While I was not concerned about my driving, I did not like the idea that I was being requested to take a test. I checked into the test and found that it was not covered by insurance. I do not understand why these doctors keep ordering all these tests that they know are not likely to be covered by insurance. All these deductibles and added costs add up over time. I found out that if I failed the test, they would report the results to my doctor and the motor vehicles department. I was willing to take this test if I was the only one getting the results, but I was not willing to take the chance with the results being sent to others. I asked friends and family how they felt about my driving and they were not concerned. That was good enough for me.

I reached out to Dr. Jordan Grafman, located at the National Institute of Neurological Disorders and Stroke at NIH, to see if they would accept me into their Semantic Dementia study. I sent all of my medical files for their review. Dr. Grafman's office got back to me and scheduled

my wife and I to come to NIH in Bethesda, Maryland for 7
days of intensive testing and procedures.

In order to be accepted they must have agreed that I
had Semantic Dementia. While Semantic Dementia seemed
better than Alzheimer's, it was starting to sink in, and it was
a bit scary. Until now, no one was sure of what I had, and
now I have been diagnosed with a progressive disease. I then
started thinking that maybe they are wrong and I will wait
for my results from NIH.

In August I met with Dr. Libon to obtain his
recommendations on what type of work I can do going
forward. Below is a copy of his letter of our conversation:

*I recently met with Mr. and Mrs. Ellenbogen to review the
findings of my recent neuropsychological examination. In the
time I spent with the family I reviewed my recent evaluation,
the prior neuropsychological evaluations, the results of the
PET scan, the results of other medical studies*

*I explained to the family that we are dealing with a primary
progressive neurodegenerative disorder. My current
diagnosis is Semantic Dementia which is one of the
Frontotemporal Dementia Syndromes.*

*The family asked me about future work. I responded that Mr.
Ellenbogen is not able to return to work because of his
dementia. I do not believe he is able to manage any type of
job. At the time of my evaluation I urged Mr. Ellenbogen to
apply for disability.*

In September 2008, I felt extremely fortunate that I
was going to the NIH. All expenses were paid for by our
government through donations for research. I would have a

staff of people working with me the whole time I was at the facility.

One new word that became very frustrating for me was "caregiver." It turns out that in order to be in the program I must have a caregiver available at all times. I learned to despise that word. I had to sign some type of release that the caregiver would be responsible for me in making decisions. I was extremely aggravated by this, but I had an interest to understand what was wrong with me.

I had the opportunity to meet with many doctors throughout my stay and they performed many tests and procedures. I cannot tell you how wonderful that was, because they spent all the time needed with me and did not rush off to another patient. They gave me all the attention needed and worked at my pace, which was a bit slow. I never felt rushed.

I did hate them for the way they treated me as if I could not make a decision for myself or take care of myself. Sometimes I even got the feeling that they cared more for the caregiver than me. I think their thought was that I would no longer be around in about eight years but the caregiver would. They really need to change their attitude on how they deal with patients. I realized that I had issues, and when I did not understand something or needed help, I always asked for my wife's involvement. It is bad enough that I am experiencing all these difficulties in my life, but do not treat me like I have completely gone out of my mind. Many test results were not released because they were experimental, but their findings did reinforce the other findings. At the end, I was supposedly going to have time to speak to the people who performed the testing, but they seemed to cut me short when I wanted to cover some of my issues. Following is a copy of the actual report from NIH.

Cognitive Neuroscience Section
Summary of Research Results

Patient Name: Michael Ellenbogen
Testing Dates: September 15th – 23rd, 2008
Introduction

Mr. Ellenbogen was examined in the Cognitive Neuroscience Section of the National Institute of Neurological Disorders and Stroke as a participant in our Frontotemporal Dementia (FTD) and Corticobasal Syndrome (CBS) research protocol. Mr. Ellenbogen is a 50 year-old right-handed male with 14 years of education. He was most recently employed as Data Transmission Analyst - his retirement was related to his current symptoms. Mr. Ellenbogen has symptoms reportedly compatible with a diagnosis of FTD – semantic dementia subtype, but at the beginning of our evaluation it was uncertain what his final diagnosis would be. He was accompanied to our evaluation by his wife Sheri and an extensive family and medical history is available from the family

This report is a summary of research data and is not a clinical neuropsychological report. No clinical implications should be made about diagnosis or therapy.

Test Behavior

Mr. Ellenbogen demonstrated excellent effort during the testing and had an excellent grasp of test instructions. During the testing, he demonstrated very mild conceptual disorganization, anxiety, memory impairment, depressed affect, and language deficits.

68

Chapter 6

General Intelligence

On the Wechsler Adult Intelligence Scale-III (WAIS-III), Mr. Ellenbogen achieved Verbal Scale subtest scores of 11 for Similarities, 9 for Arithmetic, 8 for Digit Span, 7 for Information, and 11 for Letter-Number Sequencing; his Performance Scale subtest scores were 15 for Picture Completion, 5 for Digit Symbol, and 15 for Matrix Reasoning. These scores indicate verbal and visuospatial skills that appear mixed. On the one hand, he demonstrates high to above average scores on subtests measuring verbal reasoning, task switching, nonverbal reasoning, and attention to visual detail. On the other hand, he performs poorly on subtests measuring paired associate learning, general knowledge, and working memory. On the Mattis Dementia Rating Scale-2 (DRS-2), Mr. Ellenbogen attained a total raw score of 133 that falls into the normal range.

Language

Mr. Ellenbogen's score on the Boston Naming Test was 51 out of 60 items- a score that falls into the mildly impaired range. His score of 99 on the Token Test is within normal limits. His performance on the National Adult Reading Test (NART) gave a predicted Full Scale IQ score of 84 that is mildly impaired. The patient was administered the Snodgrass and Vanderwort Picture Set and out of 254 pictures shown, he only made 13 semantic errors, had 4 no responses, and self-corrected three times. His Peabody Picture Vocabulary Test score was within normal limits. He made no errors of any kind on an Object Attribute test.

Memory

On the Wechsler Memory Scale-III (WMS-III), Mr. Ellenbogen obtained an index score of 71 for auditory immediate memory, 81 for visual immediate memory, 71 for overall immediate memory, 77 for auditory delayed memory, 88 for visual delayed memory, 85 for auditory recognition delayed memory, 79 for general memory, and 102 for working memory. With a score of 100 being average for normal volunteers, these scores indicate that Mr. Ellenbogen has mild to moderately impaired free recall with recognition memory only mildly impaired and his performance improves after a delay. Note that his working memory on this test is within normal limits.

Executive Functions

The Delis-Kaplan Executive Function System (D-KEFS) includes tests that require concept formation, reasoning, and planning. On a Card Sorting Test, Mr. Ellenbogen's performance was within normal limits. His performance on a planning test, the Tower Test, was moderately impaired. His ability to shift between two verbal categories on the Trail Making Test was mildly impaired. Mr. Ellenbogen's ability to generate questions to solve a problem on the Twenty Questions Test was within normal limits. On the Verbal Fluency Test his letter-cued fluency was moderately impaired and his category-cued fluency was severely impaired. The patient's performance on a Driving Simulator was mildly impaired and included one collision, one hit pedestrian, and a speeding ticket. His memory for billboards contained in the simulator drive was severely impaired. At the time of this evaluation, the patient was still driving. The patient's smell recognition testing was within normal limits and he displayed mildly slowed response times on simple and choice response time tests

Mood State & Social Cognition

Mr. Ellenbogen's Beck Depression Inventory-II (BDI-II) score of 9 indicates he is not depressed and that score is supported by his own self-report during the testing and interviews. On the Frontal Systems Behavior Scale (FrSBe) Mr. Ellenbogen's wife reports a modest increase in apathy and executive dysfunction since the onset of Mr. Ellenbogen's symptoms (about the same concern than Mr. Ellenbogen indicates for each of these areas of behavior). On the UCLA Neuropsychiatric Inventory (NPI), Mrs. Ellenbogen also reports that her husband appears mildly euphoric or inappropriately elated at times. The patient also endorsed a relatively high level of somatic complaints on personality testing. Some suicidal ideation is present but the patient indicates he would not carry out a suicide attempt.

Summary

Mr. Ellenbogen's overall performance on our experimental neuropsychological evaluation is incompatible with his reported 11-year history of behavioral symptoms suggesting that his diagnosis is currently uncertain.

The visual inspection of Mr. Ellenbogen's MRI scan by a neuroradiologist revealed a normal brain with no obvious atrophy. A visual inspection of Mr. Ellenbogen's PET scan indicated that he had mild reductions of glucose metabolism in some areas of the temporal and parietal lobes in both hemispheres. Primary visual cortex, cerebellum, and subcortical structure glucose metabolism was viewed as within normal limits. These findings are not compatible with the typical course of a FTD.

Mr. Ellenbogen's cognitive abnormalities are compatible with the mild severity and pattern of abnormalities noted on his PET scan. His MRI scan was read as normal. These research findings would not support a clinical diagnosis of

71

FTD – semantic dementia variant given the length of time of symptoms, the minimal findings on MRI and PET scanning, and the pattern of deficits noted on his neuropsychological evaluation. While his history, neuropsychological testing and PET Scan point to a very slowly progressive dementia, at this time, we are unable to provide any more specific a diagnosis than progressive dementia.

I met with the patient and his family. I recommended that the patient's caregiver get supportive therapy to help her cope with the stresses of caring for the patient. I also recommended that the patient consider stop driving and consider enrolling in a day program to help him maintain both physical exercise and social interactions. I conveyed the usefulness of a brain autopsy to the family and they were provided with written instructions on how to obtain one if they wish. I also informed them about the newly established family association called the Association for the Frontotemporal Dementias and directed them to their www page: http://www.FTD-Picks.org/.

Jordan Grafman, Ph.D.

This report is a summary of research data and is not a clinical neuropsychological report. No clinical implications should be made about diagnosis or therapy.

A swallowing study was also performed by Jennifer Ryder at NIH. Below are her comments, emailed to me.

I diagnosed you with mild oral pharyngeal dysphagia characterized by a) oral partitioning of the pudding causing 3 separate swallows for 1 tsp and b) mild amounts of material remaining in your pharynx after a single swallow of thin liquids. I recommended no modification of consistencies you eat, but commented that you may need 2-3 swallows to

72

fully clear liquids out of your pharynx. Overall, it was a good result with the issues being really very mild in nature.

While all this testing was great, I was a bit disappointed in the results they gave us. Because many of these tests were experimental, they were not willing to share their results. I had to try extremely hard to obtain some of the information that may be helpful to me one day. For example, the swallow study was the first time I even had this test. It could act as a baseline for me should I ever start to experience problems and need to take the test again. That could be very useful. Based on their conclusion they thought I had MCI and leaning towards Alzheimer's. Apparently, the only way to make a true diagnosis is to do a brain autopsy which I volunteered to do upon my death. That could be very useful for my daughter and other future generations of her family.

I also feel that the driving test did not reflect a true driving experience. First, it had different things I had to perform in order to drive the car, unlike a real car. Second, I was looking at a computer monitor for long periods. The scanning of the retrace lines was kind of putting me into a trance. Keep in mind, I used to repair TV's and I tend to notice more issues on screens than the average person. I feel many people with disabilities may fail this test because it is so very different from actual driving. They really need to work on better simulators, after all there are great simulators available for flying a plane.

Now that many different neurologists had examined me, they felt I was misdiagnosed by Dr. Lindsey J. Robinson. In a way, I felt very bitter because I lost many years of my life trying to get the correct diagnosis. I asked my doctors if they were willing to contact her so they could educate her where she went wrong. While the doctors did not feel comfortable initiating the first move, they did offer to explain the details to her, if she would contact them. I attempted to reach out to her again. I let her know what the doctors had offered and that I was willing to share my new medical records with her. I was hoping to educate her, so someone else would not be impacted as I had been. She was not willing to listen, insisting that she was still right. I cannot understand why a Doctor would take such an attitude instead of being open-minded. Because my wife is in the medical industry, I have heard of some doctors that you would never want to deal with. Many were so bad, and doctors and nurses knew it, yet they still practiced. I am starting to feel the same way about Dr. Lindsey J. Robinson.

We are all human and we all make mistakes. If someone is willing to educate us, we should not be ashamed in any way. We should embrace the possibility of learning something new to improve our skills. After all, technology changes and we are only as good as the person who taught us. And some teachers are just not very good.

Chapter 7

So what do I do now

I had a lot to digest over the few months since I learned I had some type of dementia. I still did not think the doctors knew the cause. I was becoming more and more frustrated waiting to hear from the Social Security Administration. Every time I received new records, I forwarded them to my lawyer who also was in communication with Social Security. As I did more research on MCI/Alzheimer's it started to sink in what it meant. I have to tell you that it can be scary to think about.

It now seems that my wife is having thoughts about my driving. While overall, she sees that I can drive okay, except for sometimes when I am not in my own area. I may get lost, but that is no big deal because I have GPS. She keeps giving me cues while I am driving. I have to admit the driving report did not help my confidence. It does get to you over time, and I try to drive more cautiously than ever.

On December 6, 2008, I ended up having heart problems. The funny thing is that my electrocardiograms showed no ST elevation, which indicated nothing was wrong with me. Based on my description of symptoms, they decided to run further tests. My troponin levels came back from the lab and indicated that I was having a heart attack. Since I also have gastroesophageal reflux disease, I was living with chest burning symptoms for weeks. I was taken immediately for a cardiac catheterization. They found the Left Anterior Descending artery had 50% narrowing at its mid point. They thought that was my problem until they looked at the Right Coronary artery, which turned out to be 100% occluded at the midpoint. Based on the findings I should have been dead, but my heart was unusual because it had the capability of using my Left Anterior artery for blood flow to survive the blockage. They ended up placing three stents just in the Right Coronary artery. They decided to not do anything else with the Left Anterior Descending because of the added risk.

On February 2009, I met with Dr. Carol Lippa. She changed my Aricept to 10 mg. She said that I would not be able to return to work – cognitive and emotional features.

Well you could imagine, the heart attack made my lawyer even happier because I now had one more health issue. Below is a list of my health issues at that time. I have had some of these issues for over 10 years and some even longer.

Problems and Symptoms updated 3/31/2009

1 - Problems with memory and processing information. This leads to problems doing simple math, spelling, thinking, reading and retaining information. Impacts my daily life. Dr. Carol Lippa diagnosed - Mild Cognitive Impairment/ Alzheimer's

2 - Neck and lower back pain which prevents me from walking or standing a long time. Live with pain. PA Leanne Marada and Dr Michael Gratch diagnosed – Neck, multilevel degenerative changes and lumbar spine indicates degenerative disc disease scattered throughout as well as what appears to be a right disc protrusion at L1-2

3 – Allergies- Sneeze a lot, runny nose, and usually get an infection twice a year that lasts for about three weeks. Some
76

times itchy and watery eyes. Problems increase around air-conditioning, fans and dusty environment. Have difficulty sleeping because nose becomes congested. Dr. Shilpi Narula diagnosed – Allergic Rhinoconjunctivitis and Vasomotor Rhinitis.

4 - Body needs to be elevated about 8 inches, cannot lay flat on stomach or back. I get heartburn and stomach pain. Wear loose pants around waist. Dr. Louis Morsbach diagnosed gastroesophageal reflux.

5 - After standing awhile, or lifting, my hemorrhoids act up and become very uncomfortable and hurt, also bleeding. Dr. Louis Morsbach diagnosed external medium size hemorrhoids.

6 - Pain in the lateral aspect of the left leg all above the knee – Still have ongoing problem daily.

7 - I see ghosting and my vision is out of focus at times. Dr. Dennis Kwiatkowski needs further testing. It could be related to a visual processing problem, and cognitive skill defect may be in effect.

8 - Hands do not heal properly after I get a cut or abrasion – Need to get a biopsy the next time I have the problem. I was diagnosed with this when I was about 13 years old, but I do not remember the name of the disease. I was told to protect my hands and keep them away from any type of dirt.

9 - Diagnosed with mild oral pharyngeal dysphagia characterized by a) oral partitioning of the pudding causing 3 separate swallows for 1 tsp and b) mild amounts of material remaining in your pharynx after a single swallow of thin liquids. I recommended no modification of consistencies eaten, but commented that I may need 2-3 swallows to fully

clear liquids out of my pharynx. Overall, it was a good
result with the issues being really very mild in nature.
Beth Solomon, MS, CCC-SLP

10- Heart Attack with 3 stents – Dr David Boland

11- Tennis elbow in right elbow and some pain in left elbow
– Dr Gallant

12- Joint pain in right elbow and some in left elbow but not
as bad and spreads 5 inches either way, both wrists sore left
more than the right now, some soreness in finger joints at
times, was not able to raise left arm up to shoulder on
vacation for one day. Some pain in left shoulder, a few days
later in right shoulder. Problem gets worse with exercise. I
had to do less work at Cardiac Rehab. Could not move wrist,
not able to button shirt, shave or wash. Pain 7 out of 10 - Dr.
C. Michael Franklin – Rheumatology Specialty Center

Sometimes I feel I was put on this earth to test out the
medical system, because I have so many issues. I used to
complain about all the problems my mother seemed to have
because she was always complaining about her medical
conditions. My wife says this may be my punishment for the
complaining.

Because of all my health issues, I made an
identification badge, engraved with the following: My name,
medical issues, allergic drug reactions, emergency contact
phone number and contact name. Because of my heart attack,
I now carry a mini pill container, attached to the ID plate,
which contains nitro. While I am not sure these items will
ever help me, it gives me a feeling of comfort. I clip these to
my pants daily, just in case something should happen to me.

Chapter 7

Below are some issues that my wife noticed and sent to my lawyer around the same time.

One snowy morning Mike went outside to get the snowblower ready for use. He came inside and told me it was too early to start. He took off his gloves and unzipped his jacket. He blew his nose, then started zipping up his jacket. I asked him what he was doing and he told me that he was going to get started. I said, "Didn't you just tell me it was too early to start?" I had to repeat that until he understood. He got upset with me, but took off his jacket.

Mike went to two Doctor's appointments alone as I had to work. He then went to his Cardiac Rehab session. I saw him after the Rehab exercise session (it is in the hospital where I work)-he was very distressed. He said he was thrown off and didn't remember his routine. He forgot to put on his monitor, he forgot his towel on the treadmill (he had been going to rehab for almost two months at the time). He also couldn't remember the instructions from the two doctor's visits. I had to call both offices to find out what had transpired.

Mike misread the train schedule (something he is used to using) and we almost missed our train to the airport. We happened to arrive at the station a half hour early and the train was about to leave. (He didn't read the wrong column – he was checking times from Center City instead of to Center City.

We were having dinner with 5 other extended family members. We sat around the table animatedly conversing after the meal. Mike had to leave the room after a while because the noise was causing him distress and the multiple voices were causing him to lose the ability to follow any conversation. He cannot concentrate with too much environmental stimulation.

I labeled his medication holders as "morning" and "dinner." They are kept in two separate areas. He took the wrong pills anyway.

Mike loses track of conversations easily. I often need to explain instructions or repeat information that he didn't grasp.

He is uncomfortable counting money.

Often watches TV commercials multiple times and then suddenly says, "Oh, now I get it!"

Into the second week of our cruise, after going to dinner every night on the 4th floor, he argued with me because he was sure we needed to go to the 5th floor for dinner.

He has difficulty ordering from a menu, deciding between the choices – because he can't remember from one to the next in order to decide what he wants.

Was speaking to someone on the phone, I was sitting nearby and could hear the caller speaking. He mentioned something to me after he hung up – I said, "That's not what the caller said."

Just to clarify – I edit and rewrite most everything Mike writes before it is sent out to anyone else. His writing skills have deteriorated.

Mike put off scheduling an appointment to take my car for an oil change. I finally learned that it wasn't because he forgot, it was because he couldn't figure out how-too many steps to figure out- who to call, deciding what date he could go, what time – it was too overwhelming.

Argues with me about concrete issues, even after I tell him that he is wrong.

Ate steaming hot food (potato), instead of letting it cool a bit, and burned his throat. Often makes the water in the bathtub too hot.

In May of 2009, the Social Security Administration replied to my appeal and scheduled a hearing for August 25, 2009. I was very worried because I was not sure what would happen if I did not get into the program. I was concerned about our financial situation going forward. It's a good thing I had saved some money while I was healthy. I always planned for that rainy day, but this really threw me off.

On July 7, 2009, Dr. Carol Lippa wrote the following letter.

To Whom It May Concern:

Mr. Ellenbogan is under my care for treatment of a neurologic condition. He is becoming more severe and is unable to work any type of job at any level of capacity.

Because of the severe progression of this it is hard for him to focus and concentrate as he can become confused and disoriented at times. It was also suggested that he not drive.

Below are some other cognitive deficit examples that my wife passed on to my lawyer that occurred in May through August 2009.

- *Flooded laundry room-forgot he was running water in the utility sink*

- *Fell out of hammock-convinced that he could not*
- *Leaves his tools outside, after use, until he happens upon them later*
- *Tries to play golf-must have someone with him to direct him to his ball on the fairway or green-he doesn't remember where the ball went after he hits it*
- *Was trying to set up his silverware at the restaurant-couldn't remember on which side of the plate the knife and fork belonged*
- *Frequently does not understand what you say to him-you must keep explaining*
- *Took Tuesday's pills on Saturday morning*
- *Constantly turns off the TV, with the remote, when he is trying to change the channel*
- *Puts ice, at the refrigerator door, in his glass instead of water-every night!*
- *Won't dust or perform other household chores because he is afraid he will break something-he dropped a crystal knick-knack when he once tried to dust*
- *Put off making an appointment to take the car in for service-the process of calling, picking a date, and picking a time was too overwhelming*
- *Confused while watching a TV show-"All new episode Sunday" at bottom of screen. Couldn't figure out what that meant*
- *Isn't comfortable counting money-always has me double check*
- *Couldn't figure out how to get his corn on his fork with his knife at dinner*

Chapter 7

- *Took a phone call-after hanging up he said, "I don't know who that was or what he was talking about." For the last year or so-*
- *Paid the wrong credit card twice so I have been taking care of the finances*
- *Has frequent difficulty with word finding*
- *Often pauses in the middle of a task-when questioned he will say, "I'm trying to figure out what I have to do."*
- *I refill his weekly pill dispenser(he would not be able to figure it out)-clearly marked with the day of week and AM and PM, he takes the wrong pills at times*

I was now becoming concerned about how much I would be paid by the Social Security Administration. I thought I had an idea from the "Your Social Security Statement" we all receive every so often. The last statement I had was two years old. The statement indicated a disability monthly payment of $2,119.00. That was only an estimate and I figured it might only be around $2,000.00 per month. I could get by on this, but it was far from my original salary of $7,083.00 dollars per month. The scary part is that you still need to pay taxes on this money. Even worse, it is combined with my wife's salary, so I get even more penalized than if I was living on my own.

I called the Social Security Administration and they just kept passing me from one area to another. It required multiple calls to finally get an answer. I had to wait for someone to run a report so they could quote me the figure. I was quoted $1,451.00 per month. That number was so different from my previous documentation. When I questioned why there was such a major difference, they tried to tell me that the "Your Social Security Statement" form sent each year is only an estimate. The person also went on to say that most people who end up qualifying always get a lot less.

I became extremely upset because that amount would cause me financial hardship. That was like making $8.36 per hour, which was far from my $40.86 per hour. I was very upset for the next few weeks until I met with my lawyer at the Social Security hearing. It turns out those idiots gave me the wrong numbers and he had a paper with the correct dollar amount which was $2,323.00. That made me feel so much better. The moral of this story is to not deal with those people, because they have no idea what they are doing, and only create roadblocks for you. Speak to your lawyer about your concerns if you have any.

Anyway, it is now August 25, 2009, and my wife and I are on the way to the hearing. We are both very nervous and concerned that I will not be approved. We have never had to deal with anything like this. I was concerned that I would not say the proper thing when I needed to because my mind did not work right any more. When we arrived, the lawyer explained a few scenarios that may occur. My stomach felt like it was turning because I was nervous. At one point, I think my lawyer was having difficulties with his laptop and was concerned on how he would access his files needed for the hearing. I think I almost went into panic mode, but I was doing everything possible to keep myself controlled.

It was our time to go in and our lawyer went in first. Within a few minutes, he returned and said not to worry because they have decided to rule in my favor. He said he had to go back to finalize everything with the judge. About an hour later, the hearing was over and I finally felt relief, with no more pressure for the first time since I stopped working. They were going to follow up with the ruling by mail.

On October 6, 2009, I received the Social Security Administration decision, which said "Fully Favorable." The sad part of their decision is, it was not based solely on my memory and processing issues. They had to take into consideration all of my other health issues along with the existing job market. There is no way I could have performed a job today, but it is sad that these people thought I could. I guess I should consider myself lucky that I had other health issues and a good lawyer. That kind of sounds stupid that I wished to have additional disabilities, but where would I be if it was not for that? The judge also recommended a representative payee should be appointed to manage payments in my interest. While I still made my own decisions I did not like that someone was telling me that someone had to take care of my financials. I had already given up my responsibilities to my wife to handle all the financials for the home. They were concerned that I would take the money and just blow it.

It took repeated calls from me and the lawyer until I received the back payments 6 months later. I received the first S.S. payment in October 2009. The back payment was issued February 2010. I thank God that this is all over. I have enough things to worry about without the aggravation they have caused me.

Sometime around October 2009, I met with Dr. Carol Lippa. I was taken off the Aricept because my sick feeling symptoms were not getting any better. I was switched to Namenda 10 mg. I was also experiencing other issues at that time. I was losing interest in many foods and did not feel like eating. I was also having more difficulty sleeping. I think I may have been depressed at times. I also had other issues which I wrote down, so I would remember to speak to the doctor about them. Every time I go to this doctor, I first meet with a medical student. It was frustrating because they would ask some things that should already be known, and they did not always do a proper exam. In the past, Dr. Lippa would redo some of the test, but most recently she just relied on the students. They would ask me if I had questions for the doctor, but they could not answer any of them. When the doctor came in this last time, I tried to get answers to my questions, but I was rushed out of the office without getting the opportunity.

This doctor was located over an hour away from home and my wife always had to take a day off from work just to be there with me. I was very aggravated that day because of the way we were treated. We made a new appointment for some time the following year. My wife was present and she entered it in her calendar. They also gave me two appointment cards for two different doctors at her office. When I got home I realized that the dates were for the wrong doctors. I called and they checked their records. They said that what I had was correct. Later on, I canceled the appointment with one of the doctors but kept the other.

One day I received a reminder call for my appointment. The appointment was wrong according to what we had. It turns out that the original discrepancy I had called about was something they should have caught. Their people were quick to point out that it had to be my fault. Luckily for me, my wife also wrote on her calendar what the secretary had said and it matched with my thinking. This was the second time this has happened. It would now take about 5 months to get another appointment. I escalated this matter to the office manager and she was going to check to see if they could get me in sooner. The office manager never called back, so we switched to another doctor closer to home.

86

Chapter 7

While she may be a great doctor, they need to give some respect to their patients.

In November 2009, I had another MRI without contrast. The results were read as normal. I also had another PET scan and the impression is as follows:

Diminished metabolic activity throughout the posterior parietal cortices and temporal lobes, left greater than right. Similar findings were present on the previous exam and in the appropriate clinical setting suggest Alzheimer's dementia, without significant progression.

While I may have a progressive dementia, mine seems to be taking a different course. This is a good thing on the one hand, because I will have many more years to live. On the other hand, it scares me that when I am no longer functioning, and need the full assistance of others, it will take a much longer time to die. I do not want to become a burden to my wife and family. I have been fortunate enough to save a few dollars that I hoped to use for my wife and me at retirement. I do not want to see the money wasted on me and possibly affecting my wife's life.

I went out to many web sites looking for some possible direction on how to deal with death or suicide. I was very surprised that the Alzheimer's and FTD organizations had nothing to deal with the topic. While they may be trying to be politically correct, I think their readers would like to see some options on this topic.

I finally came across the site (http://www.finalexit.org/) run by ERGO (Euthanasia Research & Guidance Organization). This site talks about how to end your life if terminally ill and the suffering is unbearable. This is a very touchy subject and I tried to speak to my wife about it, but she just did not want to discuss it.

She feels that she would have no problem taking care of me all the way to the end. Since she happens to be an RN she feels she could take off for a year to become my private nurse, if and when I became bad. But I have many fears of reaching that point in my life. First of all, I do not want to be remembered as the person who could no longer talk or take care of himself. I want to leave this world with dignity and not make others feel better about themselves because they kept me around to the end. I do not want to frustrate and burden their lives any more than I have. While we have had a great life, those are the thoughts I want to leave my wife with. I also hope that she finds someone new in her life so she can move on. My daughter lives in another state and I do not want her to feel obligated to move back, close to home, just to help her mother. I do not think my wife realizes what a major undertaking this is. While she may be good at what she does, she cannot handle this type of pressure.

Then of course, I do not want to suffer and be tortured for the rest of my life. There are many times, on a daily basis, when I am not always clear on what I need to do to make myself more comfortable or not suffer from pain. In the middle of the night, while sleeping, I become uncomfortable because I'm hot, so I flip the covers off my feet and feel so much better. A few hours go by, and now my feet are cold, so I replace the blanket. Now imagine that you are hot, and there is no way to remove that blanket. I would go crazy because I could not do that and would suffer. That is exactly what would happen if I could no longer do or think for myself.

My wife seems to think that those types of issues would not bother me. Who really knows? However, I do not want to be the one to find out and suffer. Sure, she can want to think it will not happen, for her peace of mind, but what about me?

Chapter 7

Let me give you another example. I have major allergy problems and I constantly have a postnasal drip. Its major impact to me is at night and I frequently wake up gagging and coughing in an effort to clear my nose and throat. Sometimes I can waste 45 minutes before I finally resolve the issue. I actually suffer today and feel tortured at times. Can you imagine if that happens to me and I cannot let someone know what's bothering me and cannot do anything for myself. That frightens me to no end. My allergist has run out of options with me. This problem has really become much worse this year.

One last example. I am particular about how my pillow feels when I go to sleep. I like it to be very fluffed up. Usually once during the night I tend to flip it so that I get the fluffed end again, and it feels so much better when I do that.

People may tell you to wait until it gets worse, but they are wrong. You need to make plans when you are still able to think clearly. You must figure out a method so you know what to do when the time comes. The scary part for me is knowing when the right time may be. You do not want to go earlier then you have to, but you do not want to wait until the point where you may not be able to decide to do it, or remember how to do it. That is why I am a true believer in assisted suicide. It would be nice to let someone know my wishes far in advance, and when we get to that point they would instruct me on what I had to do. This way, my family and I could get the most out of my life without question.

We have a game room in our house. Unfortunately, many of those items require constant maintenance. The last time I had a problem with one of my pinball machines, I spent over two hours trying to figure out why it was not working. After making all kinds of adjustments, I finally determined that one of the balls just fell out of play, and was on top of the plastic mold. This should have been a five-minute fix. I am lucky I didn't cause more problems. I am now trying to sell the games because I am no longer able to maintain them.

In December, my wife and I went to help my daughter settle into her new home. I needed to install three ceiling fans. I installed many ceiling fans in the past. This time was very different. While I was trying to install the fan, I was having some difficulty. My wife and daughter were frustrating me, because they kept yelling and trying to tell me what I should do next. While I did need their help, I needed time to think about what I planned to do and needed to work at my own pace.

I could tell my wife was starting to become depressed over the last few months because I now had a diagnosis that was terminal. Between her job and everything else in her daily life, it was becoming too much for her. I tried to go with her to counseling, but she did not really seem to want to go. She had gone twice and decided she did not need to go. I thought she might be able to get help, like I did, because it felt good for me to speak with someone. I also think the counselor we had was not the best fit, compared with others I had spoken with in the past.

When I informed my mother and sister of my diagnosis, they seemed to be in denial. Every time I spoke with them, they tried to convince me that I did not have a progressive disease. My sister even went to the point of contacting doctors outside the U.S. and insisted that my doctors were wrong. I cannot tell you how aggravating that is when all these people are trying to make it sound like it was not a big deal.

90

Chapter 7

Another thing that became very frustrating was the way my mother was starting to treat me. I used to do some minor repairs for her from time to time. The last two times, I think I just made things worse and I tried to tell her that I was not the right person to ask for repairs any more. My mother still asked and I just could not say no, and again I probably did something wrong. She finally realized not to ask me to do things for her. Over time, she stopped counting on my advice and no longer asked. I felt that I could still contribute some good ideas, but every time I mentioned something that she disagreed with, she would say things like, "It is the disease that is talking." That would frustrate me. If I spoke in a loud voice, she would blame the disease. I always talked loud and she knew it.

The past couple of years I kept forgetting to call my sister for her birthday. Last year, I even took additional steps to try to remind myself, but it failed to work. This year my sister actually had the nerve to be extremely upset with me because I did not call her on her birthday. She knew about all my issues and I was amazed that she would hold such a thing against me. I decided that our relationship was no longer important if she felt that way. It took a while before we spoke again. People around you need to be more understanding and stop kidding themselves that nothing is wrong. They need to learn that some things will not be the same any more. They should not just write you off, but should ask you about what your limitations are.

It has been over a year now that I have not been working. I keep trying to find a volunteer job where I can do something meaningful. I do not want to answer a phone or push a gurney around. I was a very good negotiator and pushed for outstanding customer service. I tried to reach out to a local hospital where I offered my services for free. They really could have used someone with my skills, but they told me that they could not use a volunteer for a paid job position. I suggested they create a new position that expanded across multiple areas. It would be unique and would not compete with another existing job. They decided not to bring me on board.

I keep my car in the garage, and many times now, I have backed out only to realize I almost hit my side mirror on the garage frame. This happens often that I notice it just after I pass by the point of impact.

In March of 2010, my daughter visited us for a few weeks. She kept her car in our driveway. One day I backed my car out of the garage and ran into her car. I was very lucky that I did not damage either car. My wife and daughter were there when this happened. My concern was that my wife might use that as an excuse to tell me to stop driving.

I used to like to tinker with electronics, but I no longer can do that because I damage what I work on. I realized that I liked playing with small engines, because you cannot damage them if you do not put them back together properly. Either they work or they do not work. I had contacted a local engine shop in my area and offered my services for free, but they thought I would get in their way.

For some reason, it seems no one is willing to give people like me a chance to use the skills they still have. Yes, I may not be perfect, and I will be slow, but I will probably be able to save the company money.

Some of the issues I deal with today are:
I used to be able to remember how to return to a destination once I had driven there before. In fact, I could get there using different routes because I had a good sense of

direction. Today I am lucky to get there with the help of my GPS.

There are times when I drive that I make a mistake. Sometimes I do not notice something or someone as quickly as I think I should. I am not sure if this is related to my condition or not. These things happen to others all the time and they are normal. If I ever feel that I am dangerous on the road, I will voluntarily give up my license. I really dread that day, because I feel like it is going to be the end of my life.

If I met someone I knew, or just met someone, I would always remember that person and would recognize them if I saw them again, even though I might not remember their name. I was never very good with names. Now I am lucky to remember their face four hours later.

I have difficulty making choices at restaurants. I cannot retain what I read on the menu, to compare it to the next item, so I can make a selection. I really have a tough time when the waiter/waitress recites the specials of the day.

Another problem is that if I eat something I do not like, I cannot remember to avoid it the next time.

I have days when I get in the bathtub and after relaxing a minute or two, I am not sure if I washed up. Therefore, I check the soap to see if it is wet, so I can figure out if I did.

I sometimes skip shaving, only to realize that I forgot when I notice my face feels scratchy.

My shaver has a red light that goes on when I should charge it. I always used to charge it regularly. Now I know it needs charging when it stops working.

From the Corner Office to Alzheimer's

I do not clean the shaver out until it is overflowing with hair and it's falling out from the shaver. I always used to clean it regularly before that would occur.

My nails are always much longer before I trim them.

I usually wash my hair 2 or 3 times a week Sometimes I go longer periods, because I am not sure when I last washed it. It even starts to feel or look dirty.

While this next thing is not bad, it is very different for me than a few years ago. I find myself, at least once a day, just getting close to my wife and cuddling with her.

I now have a fear of heights and it is very hard for me to climb high on a ladder. About 2 years ago, I went on the roof and suddenly started to panic about being there. At first, I froze and wondered how I would get myself down. The fear of thinking that the fire department would have to come was my incentive to get off.

I try to maintain a regular schedule and wake up daily at 7 AM so I do not become lazy.

It is something how the mind works. The other day I was telling my wife that I saw a boat that looked interesting. She said we had owned one of those and I asked her if she was sure. I kept trying to think about it, but I could not remember. We had four boats in our lifetime and this boat would have been the second to last.

Many people do not like computers, but I have to tell you that the computer is allowing me to still do many functions that I would not be able to do today. My spelling has gotten much worse, and Microsoft Word has improved to help me with my spelling even more. Microsoft Outlook

94

calendar allows me to keep track of all my schedules and reminders daily. I can search for files on my hard drive in seconds using Windows 7.

I still like to read these days, but do not seem to remember much about what I read. Most of what I read makes sense to me while I am doing the reading. Sometimes I lose my patience when reading long articles. I think I lose my patience in reading when I do not understand the words. Reading any type of instruction manual is very hard. I need to read the sentences over and over until I finally understand.

It is amazing how many ways I discover to work around my memory issues. It seemed I am very creative in coming up with new ideas to help me get by without others noticing my issues. One problem I struggled a lot with was keeping track of different passwords. Every company and Web site wants a password. You do not want to use the same password for all your sites because you will have a security risk on your hands. I created a system that works for me. I first came up with a system about 7 years ago that has really simplified my life. Unfortunately, I cannot share my method because my wife feels I would make hackers aware of my system and it should not be written in this book.

I would always lend things out to family and friends. The other day, I went to use a BB rifle that I had, only to realize it was not there. I tried to recall to whom I had lent it, but could not remember. I contacted all my friends and family and no one claimed to have it. I guess I can no longer do this, because of the risk of not getting things back.

I bought paint over two years ago and still have not used it to paint my kitchen. I do not know why. I just cannot do this task. I keep looking at flaws in the walls and realize it needs work badly, yet I cannot get myself to do it. I do have some fears that I may mess it up and get paint in places that I should not.

There are many other things waiting for me to get to them, but I just cannot get myself to do them. This is so different for me, because years ago, I was the complete opposite. I would not let things wait. I had to get them done as quickly as possible.

I cannot seem to do things in a timely fashion. For about a year, the water softener system in my house has not been using salt like it should. I think there may be a problem. The only way to know is by scooping all of the salt out to check. I cannot seem to get myself to do this. I keep thinking about it, but I never do it.

The other day, the garden hose reel broke. It has now been laying there for two weeks with the hose partially out. I could probably fix it if I remove the hose. I even have another one I could use if I cannot fix it, but instead it's still sitting there.

I came back from the shore with two chairs that had sand on them and required hosing down. I hesitated to use my car, because I did not have room in the trunk. After two weeks, I finally took them out when I had to take my wife shopping. I am not sure why I keep doing this. If I were being paid by someone to do something, or hired by someone, I am sure I would do the work immediately. I don't know why that should make a difference.

I am considering paying someone to paint the outside of my house and to do some minor repair work. I never paid anyone to do that in the past. I always did it myself.

Chapter 7

It is the beginning of July 2010, and I started working on this book. It is a month and a half past my 52nd birthday. I have to tell you, I cannot believe I am attempting to do this again. After having the experience of writing a book in the past, I never thought I would do this again. After giving it a lot of thought, I felt this may be able to help others, which has always been my life's goal.

The other day I met a wonderful lady from the Alzheimer's Association. She made me aware of some opportunities where I may be able to contribute my time to help the organization. She also offered possible opportunities at companies in my area. She offered to contact the company on my behalf and be there if I felt the need for her to defend my cause. It is great to know that there are others out there who understand people like me. She had lots of good information to share. In fact, I was surprised to find out that there are many younger people, around my age, who have Alzheimer's disease. My doctors seemed to imply that I was very unusual. It was also interesting to learn that most of them were very high level individuals who were able to self determine that they had some type of problems and sought answers early on. I also learned that African Americans were twice as likely to get this disease. You wonder why. It seems that I may become a spokesman for the Alzheimer Association. I may also help by representing them in Washington, as an activist. They also have some committees that sound very interesting that focus on helping others. I have to tell you that this is the first time in years that I felt that I may finally have found something meaningful to do, that will benefit others. I cannot believe that I am even considering speaking in front of a large group of people. When I was healthy, I would always refuse to do any type of speaking engagements. I was always afraid of being up front and speaking. I am now more concerned with helping others.

I got up at 5:00 AM this morning with many thoughts going through my mind. My brain felt like it was on fire. One thing that kept coming to mind was the word "caregiver." The other day this word came up again. As I think I said before, I hate and despise that word. I was wondering how others felt about that name, especially those in the early stages of dementia. Did they ever ask what patients thought before using that word? I think a more appropriate name would be "assistant." If I were referring to that person, I would say, "my assistant." Now I am not sure how those who are caregivers would feel with that change, but they should keep in mind that we are the patients. For them it is only a job name, while to me it feels like a description. I have no issues using the name if I was in the final stages of the disease, but right now, I find it demeaning.

It's funny that I just realized that I have one additional ailment that was not on the original list sent to my lawyer last year. I have a condition opposite of diabetes. I have hypoglycemia. My sugar level drops quickly sometimes if I eat sweets or too many carbohydrates. I start to feel nauseous, become jittery and shaky, and start to get the sweats. After a while, I feel like I may faint or fall down. My wife says I look pale when this happens. I need to eat something sweet quickly. The thing that works best for me is orange juice.

One issue I really have a problem with is when people talk to me I tend to not remember to take notes. I think that is because I never had to do this in the past and would always remember details without writing them down. I do not understand why I cannot get used to doing this simple task. On the other hand, there are times that I do take notes. Then I find them later on and I cannot figure out why I took them in the first place.

Chapter 7

The other day I came across an article that really scared me. It was contained in some literature that was given to me by the Alzheimer's Association. It referred to patients that had Alzheimer's and who owned or had guns in their house. It spoke about how these patients did not recognize their family member, and shot them thinking they were an intruder. While I have a carry permit, it is due to expire soon. I was going to renew it, but now I will give it up. After seeing this article, I have decided to sell all the guns in my house. It is not worth the risk and I'm not sure I will be able to make that decision if I get much worse. The only issue I thought about last night is that this may have been my way out. While it is a tough decision to give the gun up, I have to give priority to the safety of my family.

Because I want you to truly see and understand all of my issues, I will show you my actual writing skills as they are today. While my writing skills are very poor, they would be much worse if it was not for Microsoft Word, which helps me a great deal with spelling and formatting. The following excerpt has not been edited. It was the original first chapter of this book. I have since shifted the focus, but have included it here for you to view a sample of my writing before it is corrected.

About my family and me

I was born in Bucharest, Romania on May 15, 1958. At that time in Romania was a communist country. My father was a very successful high-level person who worked at a radio and television station. At my age of 4, my parents bought their way out and moved to Paris, France. They left with only the clothes they wore. The government punished people who left the communist country. We stayed in Paris, until we were granted a visas into the United States Of America. I was 5 years old when we arrived here as legal immigrants.

From the Corner Office to Alzheimer's

My father opened up a TV repair business after a few years. He had a few successful TV and appliance business over the years, until he retired do to colon cancer. He struggled for many years with the diseases until it finally took his life at age 63. He was a smart businessperson. He had great negotiation skills and a strong background in electronics. He was a great father that gave me every opportunity, even though at first, we had no money. My parents made many sacrifices for my sister and I.

My mother worked in many factories at the begging to help the family survive. She was a very hard worker ann always took jobs that paid by the piece, because she worked very quickly. This allowed her to earn more money than the average hourly worker. In the last 10 years of my dad's life, she was finally able to work in my dad's business who sold small appliance to give her something to do. She was a hairdresser by trade, but was not hired do to the language barrier. As of July 6, 2010, my mother is 81 years old. She has had a tough life as far as the last 15 years. She has Rheumatoid Arthritis, and many other pains that have made her life very uncomfortable. She has high blood pleasure that was is hard to maintain at a constant level. She also suffered from many drugs that she would take because they either made her sicker or broke out from rashes. This also prevented her from getting the relief needed.

My sister is 10 years older then I. She was healthy until she was diagnosed with breast cancer at age 33. She went on to beat it, until she ended up having a heart attack in 1994, when she was 47 years old. Since then, she had bypasses and other heart attacks. Today she can only walk about a block before being to tired to walk any further. Within the past few years, she has gotten much worse. She now ends up in the hospital often. She seems to be there every two months, do to her lungs filling up with fluids. This is due to her heart not working as it should. Unfortunately there is nothing more the doctors can do for her and she will continue to suffer this way.

She had had two children, one is 40 years old and the other is 43. The oldest one was fine until 7 years ago when she was ill with vertigo. Because of this illness, she was forced to quit her job. Her illness continued for over 5 years. She was not able to stand or walk due to the risk of falling. At home, she had to crawl around like a baby.

Getting back to me, I was overall a very healthy boy growing up. I had a skin condition that was could never be diagnosed. When I received a cut or wound on my hand, it would take months to heal. A small cut would become very red and swollen, around the area. Using

100

creams like Neosporin helped. I also had to remove the scab many times or the skin would grow over the scab and it would then become infected. I still have that issue today.

As a young boy and throughout my teens I always seemed to get in trouble for one reason or another. I was never very good in school. I could never seem to sit still. I was always doing something or talking which ended me in special classes at a young age.

When I graduated high school I went on to technical school to receive an associate's degree in Electronics Technology. While I was never very good in school and had grades in the c range. When I went, to technical school I totally changed and was very interested in the classes. My grades also changed to A's and B's. I never felt that I was smart in high school, but I definitely excelled above the rest of the students in tech school.

I originally went to school so I can repair electronics, but when I graduated, I was offer a great opportunity in data communications. In 1980, I started to have signs of lower back problems and required to wear a back brace for a while.

At my first job, I was very enthusiastic and learned a lot about telecommunications. I had also married around that time. Within 5 years I left my first job and went to work for another company were I really became very knowledgeable in telecommunications. After 3 years, I took another job with Provident National Bank, which is now PNC Corporation.

I was very fortunate because I quickly moved up the corporate ladder and held many position along the way.

I have always liked to travel. In the past 3 years, my wife and I have taken some lengthy trips, to many parts of the world. I really enjoy going to all these places and love all the activities. When I get back home, I may remember a few names of the places. After a month or two, I may be lucky to remember one or two places. We usually visit 5 to 8 places on every trip. People always ask about my trip and I cannot tell them much about it. It becomes frustrating when I cannot have conversations with others about the locations I have visited.

Today I try to keep busy by cutting a few lawns on my block. It gives me something to do, and gives me the opportunity to get some exercise. It also gives me a sense of accomplishing something.

When I cut grass, I am not as careful as I should be. I am doing better today than a year ago, but sometimes I overlook safety issues. I keep the lawn tractor in my shed, which has a vinyl mat on the floor. Most recently, when I started the tractor, I engaged the blades and sucked up the matt into them. I did the same thing a few times. I'm not even sure why I ever engaged the blades in the shed.

When I use the weed whacker I consistently hit my legs and glasses with stones. In the last two years I have ruined my glasses. I would have never scratched them in the past. Now I wear safety glasses most of the time. If I forget them, I remember if I am hit again. I also wear long pants to protect my legs. I also now wear noise-canceling headphones. If I do not use them, I really have a lot of difficulty tolerating the noise. It almost feels painful. A few years ago, I never used any type of ear protection.

A few months ago, I attended a family affair, which I had been looking forward to. The loud music was hurting my ears to the point that I was suffering in pain, and I could not hear any discussions going on at the table.

I do not know if it is my imagination, but it feels that some people that used to speak to me regularly, may not be doing it as often.

Chapter 7

I do realize that sometimes I say some stupid things during a conversation. This happens because I cannot recall many of the facts that I would like to bring up and the wrong thing comes out of my mouth. That makes me feel stupid. I really miss being able to have a great conversation on a political or news topic, but I just cannot remember all the facts. Another issue I have is I may be speaking about a specific topic and something comes to mind about something similar, I switch topics and forget to go back to what I was speaking about in the first place.

I often do not enjoy going to out to dinner with others. I find there is too much noise and I cannot hear most of the conversation. I have found it to be better to go out during the week, around 5 PM. This makes a big difference in many places because I am able to hear what is going on.

I do not think that they still make these, but I think other similar devices like them can be useful for anyone with dementia. I used to have a Texas Instruments PS-6860Si. This electronic organizer allowed me to store phone numbers, appointments and notes. It turned on quickly and allowed me to see information immediately. They need to make a device like that today that is simple to operate and can sync up with your computer.

It is a good thing that I finally do not need to see doctors as often, because I probably could not afford it today. My wife's health plan not only increased the annual cost for the plan, but it also increased all of the other costs associated with drugs and co-pays, along with other new limitations. It seems to me that people, going forward, will delay getting medical care due to the added costs. One day this will hurt companies when they lose employees due to poor health conditions. This will happen because it will be too costly to address what would have been a simple health problem when it could still have been managed easily. This kind of stuff scares me because I no longer have the option to switch to my employer's insurance plan, since I no longer work. You would think a hospital would know better.

Today I asked my wife if my next-door neighbor always had two doors at the back of the house. She said yes. We have lived here for about 19 years now.

My wife takes care of dispensing my pills. I still order them, when she asks me. Today she gave me a bottle of pills to order that were very distinctive looking, and I asked her if I take these pills. At the same time, I was taking my morning pills and noticed that they were the same as the ones in the bottle. What I truly find amazing is how some things I can remember and other things I cannot, even if my life depends on it.

After taking care of all the household financials for all these years, it has become extremely aggravating to watch my wife do it. I used to balance everything to the penny. I always made sure to follow up on every bill that was not the usual balance. I always made sure to follow up on rebates and any other savings that would improve the bottom line. I was always timely and ensured I was getting the most interest for my balances. She does it so differently that it just frustrates me to no end. There are times that I just want to jump in there and take it over again, but I realize that I cannot do it alone. There are many credit and saving opportunities that will never be taken advantage of again.

I have many troubles with words like these: where – were, there – their, hear – here, peak - peek There are many others that I cannot think of at this time. I am always using them in the wrong place. Many words I do not recognize or I look at one and think it is not a word. I also have issues with when to use the period (.) and colon (:), in reference to money and the time.

One of my long-time friends sent me directions to his new house. Unfortunately, his home was not listed in the GPS. I found the directions to be a bit overwhelming, and I was concerned that I may get lost. I don't currently have a cell phone. I am actually in the process of getting one, which will come in handy for times like this.

I know people around me expect less from me now, but somehow I need their help to rebuild my self-esteem. I am pretty sure it is very low at this time. I think if they help me build some of that up, I may do better.

In closing, I am not sure how long I will live, but I hope not to miss my daughter's wedding, and seeing her first child. I would love the opportunity to spoil that child. I hope I will be able to be trusted with the child.

When I pass on, I want my family and friends to listen to this song and think of me. (Tina Turner and David Bowie – Tonight) Every time I think of this song, it makes me think of my wife, daughter, family and friends. I become very emotional and I get choked up. Many songs make me feel this way today, but not like this song. I have become very sensitive to songs, TV programs and stories that trigger my emotions.

I have accumulated many new items over the past year from a past project. While I do not need these items, I cannot seem to get rid of them. They are taking over parts of my house and I do not know what to do. I almost feel like one of those people that hoard everything, but I know I am not. I recently did throw away many items from past work positions, that I no longer need.

From the Corner Office to Alzheimer's

I have to tell you a funny story. First of all, I did not own a cell phone until yesterday. Because of my issues, my wife and daughter insisted on getting a phone so they can reach me when they need to. I can also use it if I get lost when I am driving. I did have an opportunity yesterday to hear it ring. Today I went to the ATM and was in the middle of a transaction. All of a sudden, I heard music playing and I was trying to figure out why the ATM started playing the music. Luckily for me my wife was with me, and she told me to answer the cell phone.

I am not sure if this is a song, but that was my goal when I started writing it. I was trying to write something for my wife to have after I am gone. I think I started working on it in September, 2006. I think it was finally completed about 2-3 months ago. A friend told me it was incredibly moving. He also thought it made a good poem. Besides the goal to have this book published, I would also like this song to be sung by someone famous, and a copy of the record to be given to my wife and daughter. If I had a choice, it would be Celine Dion. Talk about high hopes. I would also like to see it as a poem.

Keeping the course

My gorgeous love, I don't know where I'd be, if it wasn't for you
When I strayed, the wrong way. You were always there for me.
When others didn't believe in me, you always knew, and stood by me.

We were so young then, but we did not care, we did not care.
When I thought I was untouchable, but you knew better.
I tried to make you go astray, but you were so much brighter in that way.

Where would I be, Where would I be, Where would I be without you, my love.

The longer we knew each other, the more we became inseparable.
While I've had, regrets, for some of my actions, I have none for meeting you.

106

Chapter 7

We succeeded in creating our course, because you always watched over me.

We finally married, after all those years, beating the odds, of even our parents.
My life had really changed, because I now had, the gem of my life.
We began our new life, after moving to our new home.

Where would I be, where would I be, Where would I be without you, my love.

We met new long term friends, which had the same long term ideas.
One by one, our friends added new life, as we saw each other's families grow.
While we were still on course, and knew our next heading.

Five years later, you made me happier than ever.
You gave new life, to our beautiful little girl.
We made our parents so proud and happy, which put us right on course.

Where would I be, Where would I be, Where would I be without you, my love.

As we went through some sad times, Jamie's growing, helped us cope.
She turned out to be, better than one, could have hoped for,
21 years later, she graduated CMU, and I was no poorer, because I had the both of you.
Now prepared, to meet her challenges, she started her own new course.

35 years later, we're doing so well, as we moved on the course.
Who knew then, that my sweetheart, would become my daughter's mother, and lovely wife.
Then all of a sudden, we were hit with the surprise, of my health, not so fine.

Where would I be, Where would I be Where would I be without you, my love.

While Jamie upset me at times, she made me a proud father, in the way she turned out.
Her intelligent mind, was set in her ways, as she adventured, her new course.
She made us so happy, when she moved in her house, it just reassured us, she was dead on her course.

But I cannot complain, because I had you and Jamie, and a wonderful life.
Don't look back, keep up your smile, and stay the course.
One day, in the distant future, we will collide, and start our second course.

From the Corner Office to Alzheimer's

Where would I be, Where would I be, Where would I be without you, my love.
Where will I be, Where will I be, Where will I be without my love.

It is now September 12th, and I have to tell you it has been an exciting few weeks. The Alzheimer's Association had given me information on a few places where I may be able to volunteer. It's been hard to find something meaningful to do because I want to still make a difference in this world. I have been searching for something to do for over two years and I think I found my calling. I met with Cass Forkin, the founder and executive director of the Twilight Wish Foundation. This organization believes it's time to say "thank you" to seniors by bringing smiles and joy into their quiet, humble lives. They do this by honoring and enriching the lives of deserving seniors through a wish granting program. The Twilight Wish Foundation is a 501(c)(3) non-profit charitable organization, based out of Bucks County, Pennsylvania. This organization was started in 2003, and now has many chapters across the United States. Many of our seniors have given so much, yet they are forgotten.

While I have many difficulties, I will be a major asset to this cause. I had the opportunity to attend my first meeting the other day. I have been added to the board to help in deciding who gets their wish, and to help in the process of making the wish come true. I had the opportunity to work on my first wish the other day. Unfortunately I could not work on this task too long because I was preparing for our cruise. I have to tell you that it felt great to know that I was using my skills again to try to make someone happy, that really needed it. The wish I was trying to fill was for a 78-year-old woman who lived on a 9-acre farm and had run in to financial difficulty over the years. Her husband had passed away in the last few years. She used a golf cart, which gave her the independence to get around the farm and do her chores.

108

Chapter 7

Unfortunately, the batteries died and she was unable to get around. She felt this would be the end of her independence and made a wish to have her golf cart batteries replaced, because she could not afford them herself. I was able to reach out to multiple companies in the area to ask for their donation to help. I don't know how this will turn out since I have turned this over to someone else at this time, while I go on vacation.

I have many concerns about the people I will be working with, because I do not want them to think that I am an airhead. At our next meeting, I plan to read the letter below, so I can be upfront with the staff and make sure they clearly know my issues and limitations.

I just wanted to let you know that I have been diagnosed with Alzheimer's. I am not telling you this because I want you to feel pity for me but because I want you to understand some of the challenges I face in doing this job.

I have to tell you when I attended the last meeting I was overwhelmed because I had a lot of difficulty trying to put all the pieces together of all of your conversations. My processing speed is slow, so while I may hear what you say it does not register. At times I spend much time trying to recall what you just said, because of that I may miss other important facts you are saying.

I do have to tell you that it was great to be sitting in some type of meeting again and it was even better to know that I was able to try to help someone with my first wish assignment.

Most people who meet me are not aware of my issue. I have learned to hide it very well and give people a false picture of who I really am. I have learned to put up this front that I am not proud of.

My other issues are retaining information such as your names, maybe even remembering your face, loss of words, poor spelling, even two and three letter words. I can no longer do math without a calculator and it has to be very basic, I also do not retain much if I read a book, newspaper or listen to someone. I cannot memorize things but can wing it in a conversation or speech. Sometimes little things seem very overwhelming to me. I no longer understand many jokes.

But believe it or not I can still be a major asset to this organization if you are willing to put up with these setbacks. I am able to get by, by having notes around me when I speak to people.

If you want me to do something it's best that you talk to me and follow up with the file or information in an email ASAP, so I can start my work. I rely on that so I can gather my thoughts when I communicate with others. Please do not assume I understand, I really can be thick at times.

Before I send something official out, someone will need to check the letter to insure the spelling and verbiage is okay.

I can assure you I will give you and the organization 110 percent on any task I accept and will not let you down. If at any point you feel that I can no longer perform this work, I will not take it personally. I was once a high level manager and truly understand. I work very, very hard to be able to do all this, and to make up for my weaknesses.

Between this job and my work for the Alzheimer's Association, I will have my hands full doing great things that will hopefully help others.

My wife has just about completed the edit of this book, but now I have a few more things to add. It's all starting to come together. The lawyer should have their chapter completed soon. Still not sure about whether I will have a doctor complete a chapter, but I am still trying.

Great news on my poem/song. I found someone who was willing to volunteer their time in putting my words to music. Some words had to be removed because of the length of the song. It could only be about 4 minutes. I found this person by asking for help on Craig's List. This nice person sent me a first take of the song and it was very exciting to hear. I made a minor change and he is working on the final version. Many people who have heard it thought it was really good. Who knows, this may even become a hit. Once I get the final version, I will see if I can get it played on the radio and see if some big star is now willing to sing it. It's easier to let someone hear it then just giving them the words. I have to say, if it wasn't for writing this book and needing my wife to edit it, she would have never known about my poem until I passed away. I am very happy that I had the opportunity to share that with her and others while I am still around.

This week I am going on a cruise to Europe with my wife. While I have been to England, I have never been to all the other places we are going. This is my wife's first trip to Europe. We decided to go to as many places as we can while I still can. Unfortunately, there are limitations on the money being spent and how much time she can take off from work. I really love going to these places and spending the time with her. I am very happy that she gets to see these places with me. It's sad that I cannot remember them, but it's sure great to be there.

A few new things have happened to me. I was eating dinner one night and I was eating very hot sauce. It fell on my skin and it was burning and I think my wife had yelled over to tell me to get it off. I am a bit slow at times to react. I also seem to have missed my medication more frequently lately. It seems that if my routine is different on a particular day, it throws me off very quickly. My wife is constantly telling me to wait before eating hot items lately, because I try to eat it as soon as she places the food in front of me.

A couple of weeks ago I had the opportunity to go to the air show. One of the people who went with me left a lot of sand on the back seat, and the inside is very dirty in comparison to how I used to keep my car. The outside is also filthy. My wife's car was so dirty, and after many hints to me, she finally washed her own car. I really do not know what and why I have changed. I always used to have clean and waxed cars all the time. I could not stand it if they were dirty.

I have the tape roll that I use to tape boxes, and I used very frequently. This time I had such a hard time finding it, even though it was in the area I normally keep it. This is one of the most frustrating things, to constantly have to search for items and waste so much time. I do have to tell you that I was very proud of myself last weekend. One of my neighbors was trying to find a broken wire underground. I have many of my tools I used to use in my field. I offered a tool to him to use, but because the cable was buried too deep, the sound was so faint that it could not be heard by the instrument. I went back in the house and started looking around in my box of electronic test gear to see if I could come up with another idea. Since I cannot remember what I have, I need to look at everything to remind myself of what I have and what they can do. After seeing a very sensitive microphone/amplifier I came up with the idea of using the two tools together. It worked better than I could have imagined. I was really impressed with myself and so was my neighbor, who also works with electronics.

On October 5th, I just came back from one of the many trips I have recently taken with my wife. I went to Europe and had the opportunity to go to 9 different countries. On one of the days we took a blue van that shuttled about 10 people. There was also another van, that was white, which was taking another group. The doors on one were on the side and the other were not. After one of our stops, I tried to go to the white van instead of the blue van. My wife stopped me from going to the wrong van. That was a bit scary to me because I did not think I would have that type of issue. When I got home my daughter asked me which place or activity did I like the most? While I had a great time in all the places and activities we did, I could not come up with an answer. I finally told her that I just could not think of any. I felt really badly that I could not come up with an answer. Out of all the places I visited, I am lucky to be able to name 6 of the places. While on the trip, we did a lot of walking in many crowds. Every once in a while I would lose sight of my wife and become a little panicky until I would see her again.

Today, October 6th, I went to my first meeting at the Alzheimer's Association. They were forming a new advisory committee for Early Stage members. They are trying to see how they can benefit future patients and educate others about the disease. This was the first time I had an opportunity to meet others like me. It was amazing how their stories were so much like mine. Some were very moving and almost brought tears to my eyes. All of these folks were in the early stage. I am not sure I could handle dealing with people who progressed to the next stage. That scares me very much because I have some idea about how they may act. That is a reflection of what I may be one day. I just do not want to see it. I am starting to get very involved with this organization and looking to help others, and hope to make it better for the next person.

My wife and I have been to a few Early Stage Support Group meetings. I look forward to that meeting and hope to learn some new things. It's very interesting to see others who are like me. It's also difficult to be with some of those same people because they don't seem to remember much of what they say. While I do have some of the same issues, I am not as bad as them yet. It's very frustrating to be with them because the meetings are not as productive as I would like them to be. It also makes me feel bad that one day I will be just like them. One thing that really irks me about the meetings is that the coordinators are trying to fit in with the group by saying that they also forget many things and they are kind of like us. While I appreciate what they are trying to do, it does not make me feel better when they try to associate their memory issues to mine. No, they do not have Alzheimer's. Many of these people are also complaining that no one is doing enough about Alzheimer's these days and about getting the word out. I feel that we can focus negatively about this or we can do something to influence the minds of others and make a difference. I have to tell you that while I may be upset at times about having this disease, I also feel blessed that I can make a difference to help others and make this a better world for people who have Alzheimer's. The only concern that I have is things are moving very slowly and we need to move faster because I do not have unlimited time.

I finally got the opportunity to hear the final version of my song. Unfortunately, I could not use all the words due to the length of time. Below are the words to the song called "Where Would I Be." The singer is Chris Nelson, from Lebanon, Pennsylvania.

My gorgeous love,
I don't know where I'd be
if it wasn't for you.
When I strayed the wrong way
You where always there for me
When others didn't believe in me
you always know
and stood by me.

Where would I be,
Where would I be,
Where would I be without you, my love.

The longer we knew each other,
the more we became inseparable.
While I've had, regrets,
for some of my actions,
I have none for meeting you.

Chapter 7

We succeeded in creating our course,
because you always watched over me.

> Where would I be,
> Where would I be,
> Where would I be without you, my love.

We finally married,
after all those years,
beating the odds,
of even our parents.
My life had really changed,
because I had the gem of my life.
We began our new life,
after moving to our new home.

> Where would I be,
> Where would I be,
> Where would I be without you, my love.

You made me happy
Happier than ever
You gave new life to our beautiful little girl
She turned out to be better than one could hope for,
For 35 years we were doing so well,
When I found my health was starting to decline
I really understood exactly what was mine

But I cannot complain,
because I had you both
and a wonderful life.
Don't look back,
keep looking forth
Keep up your smile
And stay the course that guides us
One day, in the distant future,
We will collide and start our second course.

> Where would I be,
> Where would I be,
> Where would I be without you, my love.
> Where will I be
> Where will I be
> Without my love

On 10/25/2010, I received a call from my mother who had called about an issue with her home. I did not want to deal with it so I called and complained to my sister. My sister was questioning why I could not help out. I tried to explain but she felt that I could do more, based on her observation of me. I tried to explain, but she insisted I try. I had refused and asked her if she had read this book manuscript. She said that I never gave it to her, so I sent her a copy.

The next day she called and apologized for insisting that I help. She did not realize all of the problems and struggles I was dealing with. She had spoken to my mother and they both came to the conclusion that they were both in denial until now. Because I am pretty good in having conversations they did not think I was that bad. I am also not one to complain about all my issues unless I need to. This has now removed a lot of the stress that I have when these issues arise with my family.

The moral of the story is to insure others around you know and understand your weaknesses and struggles. Start by creating a written list of your issues. Take your time so you can think of all your issues and work at your own pace. This list will get longer as time goes on. I cannot tell you how many times I made changes to this book, but it was a lot. It frustrated the people who had to constantly edit my words and writing structure.

I know I have said this before, but I really mean it this time. People who have been reading my book have indicated to me that I keep saying that I am ending the book, yet I continue on. I am writing this entry on February 11, 2011 and I do promise it will be my last addition to the book. I have to say that this book is extremely frustrating for me to write. It has really made me realize that I cannot remember

116

what I write from one chapter to another. Below are a few more issues that I feel are important and need to let you know about. Some items I may have touched on before, while others I am adding additional information related to the topic. Sorry again if I may be boring you with some of the same comments, but they do say the average person needs to hear things somewhere around 3-5 times before it registers in your memory. Not sure if the numbers are correct any more, but you get my drift.

There is no doubt that I am losing my drive to do things. I think part of my problem may be because I forget what I should do. The other issue is I am trying to do too many things for me to keep track of. I may no longer be very good at doing multitasking projects, or projects that drag out over a few weeks. I find it best to work on a single task, that needs a single resolution, which makes it much easier to focus on the task at hand.

I am becoming more frustrated trying to write words, because I am now spelling so poorly at times that Microsoft Word does not even recognize what I am trying to spell. I also seem to have a much smaller vocabulary and struggle to find the words I need to use when speaking and writing. I keep using the wrong words and only realize it a few seconds later after saying what I want to communicate. I now need to trust Word on its selection of words like (then or than) because I have no idea on when to use them. While writing the four additional pages, I misspelled the word "can" with "ken". I sometimes laugh at myself. I don't know how I come up with these things. This part has made me feel more uncomfortable about being with people and communicating. I know most people are not forgiving of things like that and many around me still have higher expectations, because I do not come across as having any issues. I probably create some of that myself because I cannot come to terms with having many more limitations then I am completely aware of. I find myself having periods when I just start to stare at nothing for a while. I am not sure how long I do that, but I do know a lot of my time passes faster throughout the day.

I used to find it boring to have nothing to do, but lately I have been okay with that and I waste a lot of time doing many of the same tasks throughout the day. I no longer seem to be interested in reading the Sunday newspaper. I am not sure why, but I never could recall much after reading, so that may be why. I almost feel like I was still reading it all this time because it was a habit that was just hard to break. I have now been reading a book that I like for about the last 4 months. The book has 324 pages and I have about 25 pages left to read. I only read it once in a while when I am trying to waste some time. Many times I need to read the same information multiple times in order to understand it. About 50 to 60 percent of the time it makes sense. As I move on from one paragraph to another, I tend to not remember much of what I had read.

I remember, about a year ago, I had trouble falling asleep and was not interested in food that much. I was placed on Citalopram, an anti-anxiety medication. My sleeping habits changed to where I fall asleep almost instantly upon laying my head down. Nowadays it takes me a little longer, but still much better than before. I also enjoy and look forward to eating foods, maybe too much because I have been gaining some weight. I am pretty sure that I was starting to feel a little depressed when I started taking this drug, but I feel great nowadays, with no sign of depression, and I also do not get as emotional. I feel I am much calmer.

I am seeing a change in my grooming, because I do not wash my hair as often as I should. I have trouble remembering when I last washed it. I may be doing similar things with other things like outdoor jackets and sweaters, because I do not realize how long I may have worn it and when it needs washing. I do not seem to care about having scuffed shoes, where I would have never been seen that way in the past. I just hope people around me do not hold this against me if I get worse. If I should become worse I would not mind if they kindly remind me that I may need to do something. I know I have almost lost my control on this issue.

I had finally gotten rid of my guns in October of last year. I quickly regretted getting rid of them, but would do it again, based on what I learned. It's amazing how confident I was when I used to carry my gun and never felt in danger of being threatened. That kind of changed after not having guns. I now purchased a stun gun which is much safer for me and everyone around me.

I have become very frustrated in making new purchases of items like a lawn tractor, snow thrower, and shaver. I am just not sure I remember all the features and issues that I read, to be able to make a good sound decision, and that really frustrates me. I misread things like "It does have mow in reverse." I understood this to mean that the mower did not cut grass in reverse, until it was pointed out to me. It's clear as day to me now, but it was not until I was told.

Below is a letter that I was asked to write for the Alzheimer's Association newsletter, which I thought would be very helpful for both the caregivers and the patient.
As an Alzheimer's patient, I find it very difficult to perform tasks that I was once very capable of performing. Sometimes I am better than other times at doing the same task. People around me have accepted this fact and have tried to be very forgiving when I run into issues doing a task or when just

trying to remember something. I really think that people around me should challenge me more at times.

For example, many of my doctors kept questioning me about whether or not I should still be driving. This of course was mentioned to my wife, who also started wondering. I finally had a driving test a few years later. It was recommended that I no longer drive, even though I passed the test. I was almost borderline, but there was concern that I may not recognize when I become worse and could then become a danger. First of all, I have to tell you that the test they performed was not fair. I wonder how many regular people would be able to pass this test. The test also relied on me to learn new things in order to take the test. That is not fair since I have been driving the same vehicle all this time and nothing has changed. This constant talk about my driving has totally killed all of my self-esteem about driving. Every time I was in the car on the road with my wife, she constantly pointed out any mistakes I made, and her reaction time was much quicker than mine. I do realize I am a bit slower in my response time, but that is why I give myself more space between the other cars. Sometimes I am very far back or I just don't want to go around that slow car. There is nothing wrong with not feeling comfortable to go around that person. Let me do it at my speed.

I see many people on the road that I feel are so much worse than me and I wonder why they are still on the road, if I am supposedly so bad. I decided that I was going to drive to visit my daughter in South Carolina. I live in Jamison, PA in Bucks County. I was very scared to take this trip but I was trying to prove something to myself. It could have meant the end of my driving if I made a serious mistake along the way. In one day, I drove about 700 miles, with the help of a GPS in my car. The more I drove, the more I started to feel comfortable behind the wheel. A few other people on the road made serious mistakes along the way and I easily avoided a possible accident. This trip was the best thing I could have done for myself. I now have almost all of my self-confidence back and my wife no longer makes constant comments about my driving, unless I have a real issue. I have now had two close calls that required quick thinking and maneuvering to avoid an accident. In both cases, it was the other driver at fault and I was able to avoid the issues without my wife's comments. Again, it may have taken me an extra second or two to react, but I was fine.

Because of this situation, I feel even stronger than ever that it is important to be challenged. I know it may be easier for you to do something for an Alzheimer's patient because it's much quicker for you to accomplish the task, but I really believe that if you take the time to coach us along the way, we may do better in the long run. Believe me, I know it's got to be very aggravating at times, but I really appreciate it. It takes a lot of patience on the part of the helper. Everyone is different and you need to know at what point in time you should not push. It's also hard to be patient and not raise your voice at the person you are trying to help, because it will only make it worse. I am not advocating that it is appropriate for all Alzheimer's patients to continue to drive. That is a personal decision that needs to be made with input from your family and others. I am just saying that just because you have a diagnosis does not mean that you suddenly are no longer able to do anything by yourself.

The good news is, I feel like I am driving better than ever in the past 8 years. And yes, I am still doing great things for people in this world. Just yesterday, a lady who had submitted a wish four years ago was at the risk of being canceled because others could not find a donor. She required 6 teeth extractions and a complete set of full dentures. Her dentures of 30years had been causing her pain and she was in financial hardship. I was able to find a doctor and office that performs family dentistry willing to offer their services for free and pick up the cost of the material. Yes there are still good people out there who care. I will continue to focus my time on helping others as long as I can because I have had a good life. While I may struggle doing these tasks I cannot describe the great feeling I get when reaching my goals.

The one thing I am starting to realize is that I am getting worse. As of March 2, I had a follow-up with my neurologist. While the basic mental exam was about the same, I am definitely struggling in my writing and when answering the phone. My writing skills are not just impacted by spelling, but now I add extra words, full paragraphs that may not even relate to the topic. This happens because I reuse many older documents to make it easier for me. Many times I copy and paste information. My wife has seen some emails lately and it seems that I convey the wrong message. I am starting to wonder if I am hurting the business I am trying to help. If I had an administrative assistant, I know I could accomplish a lot more, but I am not sure how much longer I can continue.

When someone calls and asks me for information related to something I originally called them about, I become very nervous and stressed out because I need to find my notes so I can speak to them intelligently. I cannot talk and find the information I need to discuss, and I start to panic, which makes things even worse. The whole problem is that I am trying to come across as a normal person and I start saying some wrong or stupid things, to try to keep the conversation going while I am trying to find the information. I definitely cannot do any type of multitasking. While I was once great at that, I cannot even do a single task with perfection. The neurologist just added a medication called

Razadyne 8 mg. For the first month I will only be taking 4 mg. I really hope this will make a difference.

I was really considering buying a used boat with dual engines, but all these issues have made me take another look at whether I would be able to handle the boat. I have come to the tough conclusion that I probably will not be able to handle the boat, especially under any kind of stress. A boat requires your mind to do many multitasking thoughts in order to properly drive it. It is very different than driving a car. The worst part of it is that I would have to learn the new features and controls and would have much difficulty in close quarters, where you are under a lot of pressure. It would be very easy to handle on the open water, but I have to think of the safety of my guests and others on the water. I may look into a simple single engine boat that is about 16 feet long as a compromise. I have to tell you it is not easy to try to analyze yourself and come up with a decision, especially when it works against what you would really like to do. Believe it or not, I have enough trouble driving my new lawn tractor. It is not because it is complicated, but because the controls are different from what I had before. I make many mistakes with it. Doing new things is hard to learn, no matter how easy they may seem to be.

I would like to be remembered for influencing change in many of the largest corporations, and helping others.

Chapter 8

What your doctor should do for you

As a patient with Alzheimer's, I was very aggravated because I relied on doctors to determine what tests I needed to take. I had no idea of the benefits or importance of these tests. It was also frustrating because I did not know to ask for certain tests that may have helped to diagnose my problem sooner. Because of these issues, I reached out to Doctor Oscar L. Lopez, MD, a Professor of Neurology and Psychiatry, to provide information for readers of this book. He is Director, Alzheimer's Disease Research Center at the University of Pittsburgh School of Medicine in Pittsburgh, PA 15213. Below is his biography.

Oscar L. Lopez, MD. Professor of Neurology and Psychiatry, Chief, Cognitive and Behavioral Neurology Division, Director, Alzheimer's Disease Research Center, University of Pittsburgh.

Dr. Lopez' primary research interest has focused on the distribution (incidence and prevalence), behavioral manifestations, risks, and long term outcomes of dementia, especially Alzheimer's disease and human immunodeficiency virus (HIV) infection. His key objectives have been to identify clinical or genetic factors that modify the natural history of dementing illnesses. Dr. Lopez has published classic papers examining the patterns of progression of all clinical forms of Alzheimer's disease. Moreover, he has also demonstrated the effect of psychiatric drugs, and dementia medication on the progression of Alzheimer's disease. Dr. Lopez has conducted a large scale study in the clinical diagnosis of mild cognitive impairment (MCI), and he is the Principal Investigator of the NIH-funded grant "Predictors of Alzheimer's Disease in Mild Cognitive Impairment".

With respect to Alzheimer's disease and related dementias, Dr. Lopez has conducted large scale studies in the clinical diagnosis of Alzheimer's disease and vascular dementia, and he has published the first integrative overview and outcomes of the clinical diagnosis of Lewy Body Dementia, which directly addressed the controversy regarding whether this neuropathological entity can be identified ante-mortem, especially when it coexists with Alzheimer's disease. Dr. Lopez has published the first study that linked the presence of Lewy bodies in the amygdala to the development of major depression in Alzheimer's disease patients. In addition, he is a coauthor of the revised guidelines for clinical and pathological diagnosis of Lewy Body Dementia. Dr. Lopez is currently the Director of the Alzheimer's Disease Research Center of Pittsburgh. This is a multi-disciplinary resource which oversees clinical assessments and care, stimulates dementia research and trains health professionals in Alzheimer's disease and other dementias.

Dr. Lopez is currently conducting studies, as principal investigator and co-investigator, of the factors that modulate the transition from normal to MCI and to dementia in relationship to cerebral amyloid deposition. These studies examine how cardiovascular and cerebrovascular factors create a vulnerability state for AD and neurodegeneration, and how they affect physiologically relevant compensatory mechanisms in the brain using MRI, FDG-PET, and Pittsburgh Compound B (PiB) technologies.

Dr. Lopez's publications can be reviewed through the National Library of Medicine's publication database.

Dementia work-up: What your doctor should do or order for you

Always	
Test/Procedure	**Why?**
Determine the presence of cognitive deficits (Cognitive testing)	These are brief tests that can help your doctor to identify memory, language, or other cognitive problems that affect your activities of daily living.
Determine the presence of depression	Depression is common in elderly individuals and it can cause cognitive problems. Therefore, treatment of depression can improve cognitive symptoms. However, depression can accompany Alzheimer's disease, especially during its initial stages, and in these patients, the cognitive deficits persist after the successful treatment of depression.
Blood tests	Memory and other cognitive deficits can occur in multiple systemic disorders (e.g., chronic kidney or liver failure, severe heart disease, vitamin B12 deficiency, thyroid disease, infections, emphysema). For example, low Vitamin B12

	levels and thyroid disease are common in elderly individuals. Consequently, the treatment of these conditions can improve cognition. However, Alzheimer's disease patients can also have these problems.
CT scan of the brain	The purpose of this study is to rule out the presence of tumors, strokes, or other disease process that could affect cognition.
MRI of the brain	The MRI provides better structural information of the brain than the CT scan, and it helps rule out the presence of tumors, strokes, or other disease process that could affect cognition. Importantly, some individuals cannot have MRIs due to the presence of metal in their bodies. In this case, the doctor will order a CT scan.
Optional	
Detailed neuropsychological testing	These are more sophisticated cognitive tests than those your doctor can do in his/her office. These tests are useful to detect Alzheimer's disease in early stages, especially when the brief cognitive tests are normal,

	but the person reports the presence of cognitive problems that affect social or occupational functioning.
Single Positron Emission Computerized tomography (SPECT)	This study provides evidence of decreased perfusion of the brain. There is decreased perfusion in temporal and parietal areas in patients with Alzheimer's disease.
Positron emission tomography (PET)	The PET scan provides evidence of decrease metabolism in the brain, and has better definition than the SPECT. Usually, it shows decreased metabolism in the temporal and parietal areas in patients with Alzheimer's disease.
Spinal tap	The cerebrospinal fluid in patients with Alzheimer's disease can show decreased levels of $A\beta$-42 and increase levels of tau proteins. The decreased levels of $A\beta$-42 indicate that this protein is being deposited in the brain to constitute the amyloid plaque, which is the hallmark of the Alzheimer's disease pathology. The increased levels of tau proteins indicate that there is neuronal loss (or destruction).

Chapter 8

| | However, it is not uncommon to see Alzheimer's disease patients with low levels of Aβ-42 and normal tau proteins. |
| EEG | Episodes of confusion and cognitive deficits could be secondary to seizures. The proper treatment of seizures could normalize cognitive functions. |

Chapter 9

Preparing for Disability

By John V. Tucker

John Tucker is an attorney and founding shareholder of the law firm, Tucker & Ludin, P.A., with offices in Clearwater and Tampa, Florida. Mr. Tucker is also an Adjunct Professor of Law at Stetson University College of Law. He has represented thousands of people with disabling illnesses and injuries in Disability Insurance and Social Security Disability & SSI claims for over 20 years. He frequently published articles on disability topics and lectures to other attorneys, training them on how to handle various types of disability claims. Mr. Tucker is an AV-Peer Review Rated attorney (the highest rating for ethics and skills) through Martindale-Hubbell, the oldest and most-respected attorney rating group. Avvo.com, a lawyer rating website has rated him at its highest level, "10/10 – Superb." Mr. Tucker can be reached at (866) 292-5260 or tucker@tuckerludin.com. For more information about disability claims, visit Mr. Tucker's blogs at http://erisadisabilitylawyer.com/ *and* http://tampabaydisabilityattorney.com/.

Introduction:

I am an attorney and I represent disabled people. Most people think of "Jerry's Kids" when I tell them that, but no, my clients are not physically handicapped children or the severely mentally retarded. My clients are hard working people who became ill or injured in the prime of their life. They are not retirement age yet; they are under 65 years old. They have families to support, mortgages to pay, college tuition due for their kids, and something has happened to their body or mind that robbed them of their ability to make a living. Most importantly, my clients are people wondering how they are going to pay their bills, because they can no longer work.

When Michael Ellenbogen asked me to contribute a chapter to this book, I agreed for one main reason: few people plan for life with a disability. Fewer prepare for making a disability claim someday, even when they have been diagnosed with an insidious condition like Alzheimer's or a progressive dementia. My hope is that I can help others prepare themselves for the day when they will need to look to someone else - the Social Security Administration or a Disability Insurance company - for support. In this chapter, I will tell you about the types of disability benefits that may be available to you and offer tips for documenting your disabling condition and preparing a disability claim.

Before I start, I must state an important point. There are some general things that apply to all types of disability claims. However, each person's case is unique. One person with a diagnosis may suffer from widely different symptoms or limitations than another person with the same diagnosis. Nothing can replace individualized legal advice. For that reason, though I may offer you a general outline about these types of claims, I strongly urge you to consult with an experienced disability benefits attorney for assistance with your case. Do this at the moment you are concerned that your condition will ultimately lead you to lose your ability to work. If you hire an attorney before you file your claim and that attorney helps get your claim paid without drawn out appeals, it may be the best money you ever spend.

Government Disability vs. Private Disability Insurance

What kinds of government disability benefits are available?

Everyone who works and pays Social Security taxes is paying for disability insurance under Title II of the Social Security Act. This is commonly called Social Security Disability or "SSDI" (short for Social Security Disability Insurance). In 2012, monthly payments under the SSDI program range from $1 to $2460. Some years, benefits are increased by Congress using a Cost of Living Adjustment (COLA). How much you receive is based upon a formula which uses the amount of money you reported on your taxes over your years of working.

If you are approved, it is possible to get retroactive disability benefits up to 1 year before the day you applied. Social Security has a 5 month waiting period from the day you stop working to receive benefits. To get the full 12 months of retroactive benefits, you have to prove that you were disabled 17 months before you applied. Once approved, a person can receive benefits until they turn 65 years of age. At 65, SSDI converts into Old Age/Retirement benefits, and you will get the same amount of money until you die.

To be eligible to receive SSDI, you not only have to prove that you are disabled from a medical standpoint, but you also have to have paid enough in taxes in the last 10 years before your disability to be "insured." Social Security divides the last 10 years into quarters, and you have to have received credit for half of this period of time, or 20 out of the last 40 quarters. Each year, the government sets a dollar amount to receive 1 quarter of coverage. In 2012, if you

132

earn $1,130, you earn 1 quarter of credit. So a person that earns $4,520 in 2012 would earn all 4 quarters of coverage for the year. Meeting the 20 out of 40 requirement is known as having sufficient work credits. To receive SSDI, a person must have sufficient work credits to be covered on the day they became disabled.

SSDI has nothing to do with your assets or income from investments. You can receive SSDI no matter how much you have or how much income you earn from stocks, bonds and other investments. Once you receive SSDI, it is protected by federal statute from creditors, though your other assets are not covered by that law. If you want to protect your assets, you should speak to an Elder Law or Estate Planning attorney.

Some people mistakenly refer to Social Security Disability as "SSI." SSI is actually a different program under the Social Security Act called Supplemental Security Income. SSI is an indigent benefit, meaning you have to fall below certain asset maximums (or poverty standards) and prove you are disabled to qualify. In 2012, the monthly SSI benefit is $698 for an individual.

A very small number of states offer additional benefits for disabled people. Because the vast majority of people do not have access to these benefits, I will not be addressing them here.

Tip: If you want to know how much Social Security Disability you will receive, you can a) look at the last Social Security Earnings Statement you received (though they stopped printing this in 2011), b) go online to Social Security's website to use their online estimator at http://www.ssa.gov/estimator/, or c) call Social Security at (800) 772-1213 and ask them.

Other than Social Security benefits, what types of disability benefits are available?

The only other commonly available benefits come from individual or group disability insurance. However, a person usually has to have this coverage in force before they become disabled to receive these types of benefits.

Unlike individual policies that a person may buy from a local insurance agent (which are governed by state insurance law), group coverage that you get through a private employer is covered by a federal law called the Employee Retirement Income Security Act ("ERISA"). I teach an entire semester course on ERISA to law students, and it is much too detailed to explain in a few words here. It can be a very anti-consumer law. When you have to make a claim under an ERISA plan, you should be sure to contact an attorney with extensive experience handling ERISA claims. You should be able to find attorneys that have experience handling both ERISA and individual insurance claims if you have both types of policies.

While you may be able to participate in your employer's disability plan, you likely will not be able to get an individual insurance policy that covers your Alzheimer's (or any other conditions) that already exists. Private insurance companies writing new disability policies engage in underwriting. They evaluate your medical conditions in conjunction with your age and work background to determine if you are a good risk. If an insurer knows that you have a condition, they may write a policy and quote you a premium, but they typically will exclude disabilities that result from conditions you have as the policy begins.

No matter what coverage you try to get (group or individual), do not lie or fail to tell the whole truth on your
134

application. If an insurer discovers that you did not disclose something, you will have paid premiums for nothing, because laws in every state allow insurers to cancel your coverage through a process, called rescission, when they learn about facts you failed to tell them that would have impacted their risk.

In an ideal world, you already have individual and group coverage in place when you begin having symptoms.

Tip: If you recently became diagnosed with Alzheimer's, you may still be able to get disability insurance, particularly through your employer's disability benefit plan. Many group plans have an open enrollment period followed by a 12 or 24 month preexisting condition exclusion period. After the preexisting condition exclusion period expires, a person's preexisting conditions will be covered if they did not become disabled during the pre-existing condition exclusion period. Most plans state that any preexisting condition will be covered after the preexisting condition period expires, even ones that will clearly cause a disability.

Do I get health insurance with SSDI or SSI?

If you are approved for SSDI, you will receive Medicare after a 24 month waiting period. The government does not provide any health insurance in the meantime, so if you have access to COBRA or can get on a spouse's health plan through their work, you should plan on doing so. When you finally get Medicare, you will receive Medicare Part A for free. Part A covers hospitalization. You can pay for Part B which covers physician appointments/tests and Part D which covers prescriptions. Social Security will deduct the premiums for Part B and Part D from your SSDI check. You may also be able to purchase a Medicare replacement plan (like an HMO) offered through insurance companies depending on where you live.

If you get SSI, you get an immediate entitlement to Medicaid. Medicaid does not cost anything. However, keep in mind that a person on SSI or Medicaid has to continue to prove they meet the indigent requirements of those programs (i.e. they are under the poverty line in terms of assets).

If I take an easier job with a lower salary before I leave on disability, what will that do?

If you decide to try a different job with lower pay, it will almost certainly impact the Short Term and Long Term Disability benefits you receive through your company's disability plan. Taking a big salary drop at the same company instead of leaving on disability is almost always a bad financial move. You may have other reasons to continue working that make it a good choice for you, but it will almost always cost you money in terms of disability payments through the company's plan.

If you leave the company to go take a lower paying job elsewhere, you may get no disability benefits at all if you did not apply for disability before you left the company.

Usually, a lower paying job will not impact private disability insurance or Social Security Disability. It may have an impact if you work at the lower pay rate for a long time, but the real problem you will encounter is with your company's ERISA plan that pays disability benefits.

Tip: Before you take a lower paying job or leave your employer, talk to a disability benefits attorney.

Chapter 9

**Your symptoms have started....try to get a diagnosis
from your doctors.**

Progressive conditions like Alzheimer's Disease
rarely result in disability in the blink of an eye. You, or
others around you, will start to see little things that show you
are having problems. If you start having symptoms and have
not yet started seeing a doctor to find out what is wrong, you
should certainly go to a doctor. It may take months or years
for physicians to diagnose your condition and understand
what is really happening to you.

It is important to note that a diagnosis – while not
necessary – can be crucial to any type of disability claim.
Most insurance companies and the Social Security
Administration want some type of medical label to attach to
a set of symptoms that explains what is happening. Put
another way, having a diagnosis makes it easier for insurance
adjusters and government benefit specialists to understand
what is happening to you...and to pay your claim. For that
reason alone, it is ideal to get a diagnosis from your doctor as
soon as possible.

As you will see below, just having a diagnosis is far
from proving a disability claim. It is merely a first step.
You can have any label attached to your symptoms, but the
label is not what proves you are disabled. It is how your
condition impacts you that makes you disabled. Your
symptoms and the limitations and restrictions they cause are
the proof of your disability, but most modern disability
systems require that those symptoms be reasonably tied to
some type of medical condition. A diagnosed condition
provides that first link to why you are experiencing
problems.

Tell your doctors everything that is happening to you.

Put simply, if you do not tell your health care providers about all of your problems, they will not know about all of your problems. Do not leave things out because you are at one specialist's office who you think is not treating something. Tell every doctor about every problem... including the side effects of all of your medications. A doctor may tell you they do not want to hear about something for which they are not treating you, but tell them anyway. You would be amazed at how insignificant things may actually be very important to your doctors.

Here is another tip: Be sure to tell the nurses and staff at the doctor's office too. They write a lot of the notes in your chart. They also fill out forms for doctors more often than you realize.

Remember this: no matter how many times you tell an insurance adjuster or government worker about a problem, it will not be as believable as reading about your problems in your medical chart.

Tip: Keep a journal with details about what is happening to you, and bring a copy of it to appointments with your doctors. Ask them to put it in your chart.

Your symptoms are impacting your work....consult an attorney.

In a perfect world, you should consult an attorney when your symptoms start impacting your ability to do your job. The interplay between different types of disability benefits, other laws that may benefit you (such as the Family and Medical Leave Act), and your employer's other policies can be very complex. An attorney can help you understand how all of these work together, as well as bring things to your attention that you had not thought about. An attorney can also help you begin coordinating how you put together the evidence that will prove your disability claim.

An attorney can help you even if you are not yet disabled from working. The starting point for most people is just getting useful advice. Learning how to document the problems you are having can be invaluable. A disability benefits attorney can help you put together a journal, begin conversations with co-workers and friends to help them understand what is happening to you, and advise you about the types of physicians you should be seeing from a legal standpoint.

I want to clarify that last point. Your doctors work with you to get you appropriate medical care. Though a lawyer is not your doctor, they can provide you with input about the medical specialties that are handling your medical care and review the documentation that your physicians are creating. By doing so, your attorney can determine whether the doctors are creating the type of information that insurance companies and Social Security look for when evaluating disability claims. Your lawyer does not direct your medical care, but they can help you and your doctors speak the language of the government and the insurance companies.

Tip: Hiring an attorney at this point allows them to help you control the claim process. If your attorney is with you from a time before you file any of your claims, it can reduce the chance of your claims being denied, particularly in dealing with insurance companies. Perhaps more importantly, an attorney can help you reduce the stress you are undoubtedly going to go through when you approach a point of realizing you can no longer work. Knowing that someone is there beside you who understands that process and "has your back" can mean a world of difference.

What do I want in an attorney? What should I ask them?

First and foremost, you want to make sure the attorney you speak to has experience handling the type of disability claim or claims you have. Any attorney can handle any matter just by being licensed, but that does not make them good. You want to get at the attorney's experience and skill when you talk to them. You also want them to explain how they are getting paid (see below for an explanation of the most common ways attorneys get paid in these types of claims).

Tip: Here is a list of 10 types of questions that you and your family should ask any attorney:

- Have you ever handled this type of claim (SSDI, ERISA disability or private disability)?
- *How many of each type have you handled?* This is particularly important if you have a group/employer claim covered by ERISA, because very few attorneys have much experience handling ERISA cases.
- *Have you ever handled multiple types of claims for the same client? How many times?*
- *How do you handle communications with your clients? What will you do to keep me informed about my case?*
- *Are you AV rated by Martindale-Hubbell?* (the oldest and most respected lawyer rating service)
- *Who will be handling my case? You or someone else?* It is ok if an attorney has other members of his team work with him, but your attorney should be the coach and quarterback. They think of the game plan

and put it into place. Do not hire someone who has a paralegal or another attorney do all of the work and then just puts their name on it.

- *If I want to talk with you, can I schedule an appointment on the phone or in-person?*
- *How do you want me to be involved in putting the case together?*
- *How do you get paid?*
- *Do you advance the case costs or do I have to pay for them as we go? Can you give me a range for what you think the expert fees, filing costs, reproductions costs and other case costs will total?*

If they cannot answer those questions satisfactorily or do not seem to give clear answers, do not hire them. If they do not have much experience handling the type of case you have, do not hire them. You can find someone who has the skill and talent to help you. You do not have to hire the first attorney you consult.

If you feel you cannot find an attorney and want a referral, you may call me at (866) 282-5260. I will be glad to help you find an attorney you are comfortable with who has the skill to handle your case.

Are there any online sites that I can trust to research attorneys?

Yes. Visit http://www.avvo.com/ and http://www.lawyers.com/.

Tip: You should look attorneys up online before you call them. It will help you narrow down who you want to hire, and it may give you some ideas for questions to ask.

How do attorneys charge their fees in these types of cases?

In Social Security Disability cases, most attorneys charge what is called a contingency fee. They get paid a percentage of your past due benefits if you win. If you lose, they do not get paid anything. Currently, the law allows an attorney to charge 25% of past due benefits not to exceed $6000 as a contingency attorney fee. You can also agree to pay an hourly attorney fee in these types of cases, but there is no cap at $6000. Because you can end up paying more than $6000, most people hire a Social Security Disability attorney using a contingency fee contract.

In ERISA disability and private disability insurance cases, there are three different types of fees that are charged: 1. Contingency, 2. Hourly, or 3. Flat fee. Contingency contracts in these types of cases often call for a 33% to 45% attorney fee, and some attorneys charge those fees for as long as a person is approved for benefits. The advantage of the contingency fee is that the attorney is not paid if the claim is not paid or won in court. The downside is that the fee can be higher, because the attorney is assuming more risk. An hourly fee has the upside of being cheaper if the claim is paid faster, but a downside of a much higher fee if the case is highly contested. A flat fee can work in some cases, but often has to be fairly high to cover the wide range of time that can go into these cases. Some firms will charge a combination of these fees.

By far the most common fee is a contingency fee. These fees are popular because both the client and the attorney have an interest in the outcome. Some people think they can result in a high fee, but you have to consider that few other professions get paid only if they win. Imagine if you could only pay your doctors if their care worked or your

142

mechanic only if he fixed the problem with your car on the first try.

Tip: Ask questions. Be sure you understand how the attorney fee will be paid.

Are case costs usually included in attorney fees?

No. It is common for case costs to be charged in addition to attorney fees. Attorney fees cover the attorney's time. Case costs include charges for medical records from doctors and hospitals, reproduction costs, expert witness costs for things like reports and filling out forms, court filing fees, deposition expenses, etc. Some attorneys will advance these costs and others will want you to pay as you go. It should be covered in your representation contract with the attorney.

Some attorneys will charge you for copying and postage. These are reasonable business costs, because there is a very large amount of paper involved in a disability case. However, as time goes on, more and more documents are filed or delivered electronically, and the total amount of these costs is dropping.

Tip: By far one of the largest costs in a disability claim is the charge your doctors bill your attorney for copying records. Keep in mind that you can save yourself money if you obtain copies of your medical records directly from your doctors. Physicians will often charge lawyers $1 per page or more for copies of your records, and they may give them to you for free. You may be able to control the charges from your doctors for filling out forms if you take them directly to the doctor, rather than have your attorney mail them to the doctor.

When should you apply for Disability Insurance or Social Security Disability benefits?

All too often, my clients tell me a similar story. It is about how they woke up one day and thought to themselves, "I cannot do this anymore." They knew the day would come, but when it finally happened, few were ready for it. Few people can visualize the day that a disease will rob them of their ability to work. Yet, when you are diagnosed with Alzheimer's (and many other progressive conditions), that is exactly what you have to do. When you reach that point that you are too tired of fighting your disability to keep working, the time has come to apply for disability. You may be getting pressure from your employer or your family to stop working. You may recognize that getting your job tasks done has become a herculean task. When the time comes to stop working, you want to be the one that makes the decision.

One reason why you want to make the decision is that an involuntary termination from work could rob you of your Short Term Disability (STD) or Long Term Disability (LTD) benefits. When you control the date you last work, you also control when you will be filing for disability benefits. You likely will be making these decisions with your family, but it is important to understand that you do not want to wait so long that you get fired from a job and lose benefits, if you can avoid that. You want to decide when the end of your working career has arrived, and when you do, you should immediately file for employer-based disability, private disability, and government disability benefits.

How to you apply for disability benefits?

I recommend that you file your group (employer plan) STD and LTD applications through work on your last day. All you have to do is go into the human resources office and tell them you want to apply for disability benefits. An email or a phone call may also be fine. You know your company's culture and procedures better than anyone else. But be sure to get the name of the person you speak to and note the time. If you can get the paperwork to start the process that day, then do so.

Similarly, you can call your private disability insurance company and tell them you need to apply for benefits. They will send you the paperwork or have you fill out forms online.

As for Social Security, there are three ways to apply for Social Security Disability or SSI benefits:

- **Online.** By far the easiest way to apply for SSDI or SSI is to submit an online application at the Social Security Administration's website (http://ssa.gov/applyfordisability/). There are two sections of the application for you to complete: 1. the Social Security application, and 2. the Social Security adult disability and work history report.

- **By phone.** You can call Social Security at its toll-free phone number 1-800-772-1213, and SSA will schedule an appointment to call you back

- **In person.** You can also go into your local Social Security office and tell them that you want to apply for Social Security Disability or SSI benefits. If you are not sure where the closest Social Security office is, go to the SSA's website and use their Zip Code Office Locator at https://secure.ssa.gov/apps6z/FOLO/fo001.jsp.

How long does it take to fill out application forms?

You can expect it will take you and your family around 2 to 4 hours to get together all of the information you will need to file an application for one of these types of benefits.

How long will it take to get disability benefits?

For group or individual disability insurance, an average claim decision takes one to three months. If you have to appeal, it can take longer. Many plans have waiting periods, so you have to check to see if your benefits do not start for some period of time.

For Social Security Disability or SSI, do not be surprised if you have to go through two appeals and attend a hearing before an Administrative Law Judge. Unless your condition is very advanced or you have other disabling conditions in addition to Alzheimer's, it is unlikely that you will get approved on the initial claim. An initial application typically takes 60 to 120 days to decide. The first appeal is called Reconsideration and it can take a few weeks to 90 days for a Reconsideration decision. The next appeal is a Request for Hearing by Administrative Law Judge, and that can take over a year waiting for that to be scheduled. In total, these appeals can take two to three years in some locations around the U.S.

After you apply, do not stop seeing your doctors.

The number one problem people have with disability claims of all types is that they stop getting regular medical care, particularly after their doctors tell them they cannot do anything else to help them. All of the disability systems in the United States require reasonable and regular medical
146

care. Even if you are going to a physician to record what is happening in your life, it is valuable to your disability case. Your doctor may not see the reason you are coming in since they have nothing new to help you, but failing to see a doctor for a significant period of time tells decision makers at SSA and disability insurance companies that you are not having problems any more. Do not fall into that trap. See your doctor(s) at least every 2 to 3 months and tell them about all of the problems you continue to have.

Claim forms....Make sure they get done on time and done right.

One of the most annoying parts of filing any disability claims is the onslaught of forms you will face. You and your family will need to stay on top of these forms. Some will need to be completed by you (or for you, depending on your condition), others by your family. Other forms will need to be completed by your doctor.

It is horrible to feel like your life has been reduced to some one or two page forms with little spaces to write answers to questions. Remember: you are not limited to the spaces on the form. You can attach other paper. So can your doctor.

The forms your doctor complete are likely to be the most important in your claim. I encourage you to offer to pay for your doctor's time in filling out any form. It may cost you several hundred dollars, but it will set you apart from the patients that expect doctors to spend their valuable time filling out forms. Keep in mind, doctors are overrun by paperwork, nearly all of which they do not get paid to do. If you offer to pay your doctor for the time it takes to document your restrictions and limitations, it may be the best money you ever spend.

Tip: First, do not think you are limited to the small spaces on forms. Attach another page if you need to. Second...and more important....the worst thing you can do to your claim is generalize your answers. Do not say, "I can't sit." Everyone can sit. The real question is how long can you sit and why you can only sit for that long. So, explain things in detail and give specifics about your restrictions and limitations. Ask your doctors to do the same thing.

What kinds of evidence can I submit in my disability claim?

You can submit nearly any type of evidence you want in a disability claim. Medical records and the forms your doctors fill out are very common, but you are not limited to that. You can have family and friends write letters about what they have observed. You can have your priest or rabbi tell the decision maker about the changes they have seen in you. You can send in photographs of things that depict the restrictions and limitations you have.

Just remember: disability decision makers need specifics. If you have a friend or your priest write a letter, you do not want to send in a character reference. You want to have them write about things they have seen with their own two eyes that would explain how you could not work or could not attend work 5 days a week. Anecdotes or stories about their experiences with you could be compelling if told in detail to show how your condition causes you problems.

One final point: Nothing is more important than documenting your limitations and restrictions.

You may see forms from insurers and Social Security that do not ask doctors for restriction and limitation
148

information. Other forms will be very detailed inquiring about how your condition limits you. If you do not get a form asking for detailed restrictions and limitation information then it is not important to document. Nothing could be further from the truth.

Without good, specific documentation of the ways your condition limits and restricts your activities, you will not win your claim. Period. You can never assume that everyone knows what Alzheimer's or any other condition does to someone. In fact, you should assume the opposite. Assume that no one knows….and it is your job (or your attorney's) to tell them.

One reason why insurers in particular do not ask for the specifics about your restrictions is that your failure to tell them you have restrictions is an easy way to deny a claim. The same applies to Social Security. In both systems, specific notes or comments on forms describing how limited you are, or how you are restricted from working, likely will determine whether you get paid.

Some of the limitations and restrictions to make sure your doctors understand include problems with:
- Concentration
- Memory – short term and long term
- Following directions
- Following through on things you start
- Losing focus
- Being able to convey an idea orally and in writing
- Interacting with others, particularly co-workers and supervisors
- Activities of daily living (toileting, bathing, feeding, clothing, etc.)

- Maintaining a schedule or getting to appointments on time
- Doing tasks at the required pace (think productivity, like the old "I Love Lucy" show where Lucille Ball is having problems on the assembly line)
- Unanticipated problems that cause you to get off track or stop functioning
- Unpredictable symptoms….how things will happen and you have no warning
- The impact of stress on your condition

The more specifics your doctors use to talk about these and other problems you have, the better your claim will go. If they explain you can only focus for "5 minutes at a time, followed by a rest of 1 hour" that is much better than saying you have "some problems with focusing on tasks." In other words, you want to tell your doctors specific examples of your limitations so they will be able to rephrase your examples into limitations and restrictions.

Some doctors think that if they simply write "no work," "cannot work," or "disabled" in their records, that is enough. It is not, unless your condition has deteriorated to the point of being so obvious from reading your records, that no one could deny your claim. I have been representing the disabled for two decades and I have never seen that case. Get your doctors to write specifics about how your condition and symptoms limit you.

Tip: Of all the tips and tricks I can give you, the comments in this section are by far the most important. Re-read this section. If you focus on getting these kinds of details about your condition(s) documented by your physicians, it will help you more than anything else.

150

Chapter 9

Concluding Thoughts:

Do not be afraid to ask for help....from your family, friends, your doctors or an attorney. If you are facing the prospect of filing a claim for disability in the future or are dealing with one now, your stress level can go through the roof. People like me get paid in part to help others reduce their stress, by giving information and helping you complete the claim and the legal side of things.

If you bought your own disability insurance or participated in your employer's plan, your current condition is why you have had that coverage for years. That is why you got the coverage to begin with. The same goes for Social Security Disability. It is a benefit you have a right to get, because you have paid into the system for years.

Just remember: few disability cases are slam dunk winners. You have one chance to get your claim right. Rely on your friends, family, doctors and legal counsel and make your claim matter, by documenting your claim right and getting paid.

Ten Takeaways about Disability Claims:
1. **Tell your healthcare providers (and their nurses and assistants) everything, including all of the side effects of your medications, and get diagnosed as soon as possible.**

2. **Just having a diagnosis does not mean you are disabled. Disability claims are won because you are restricted or limited by your condition(s) and you have documentation about your restrictions and limitations.**

3. Your doctor has to do more than write "disabled" on a prescription pad. They have to specify what your restrictions and limitations are in their notes, on a form, or in a letter.

4. If your doctor will not give an opinion about your restrictions and limitations, get a new (or an additional) doctor that will. It is that important.

5. You can write your limitations and restrictions down until you are blue in the face....if a doctor does not put it in writing, your words will have little value.

6. You win a disability case by showing that your restrictions and limitations would keep you from attending and doing work.

7. If you would miss more than 3 days of work per month, most vocational experts would testify that you are unemployable, because an employer would not hire you. You need to figure out how to explain why you would miss more than 3 days of work per month.

8. Do not underestimate how important your medication side effects are to a disability claim. Every time you see a healthcare provider, tell them how medication side effects limit or restrict you.

9. Do not keep things to yourself. Discuss the problems you are having at work and your restrictions and limitations with friends and co-workers. They may be able to help you document your problems later.

10. Hire an attorney with experience handling Disability Insurance, ERISA Disability, and Social Security Disability benefits <u>before</u> you file your claim.